Paediatric Hepatobiliary Disease
(Choledochal Cyst)
With Paediatric Drug Dosages and MCQs

Paediatric Hepatobiliary Disease
(Choledochal Cyst)

With Paediatric Drug Dosages and MCQs

Dr. Rahul Gupta

MBBS, MS (General Surgery), MCh (Paediatric Surgery)

Senior Resident, Department of Pediatric Surgery, SMS Medical College, Jaipur
Ex-Asstt. Prof. Paediatric Surgery, NIMS University Medical College, Jaipur

Dr. Shyam Bihari Sharma

MBBS, MS (General Surgery), MCh (Paediatric Surgery)

Prof. Paediatric Surgery, NIMS University Medical College, Jaipur
Ex-Prof. and HOU, Department of Paediatric Surgery, SMS Medical College, Jaipur

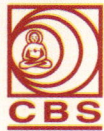

CBS

CBS Publishers & Distributors Pvt. Ltd.

New Delhi ï Bengaluru ï Chennai ï Kochi ï Mumbai ï Pune
Hyderabad ï Kolkata ï Nagpur ï Patna ï Vijayawada

ISBN: 978-81-239-2696-4

First Edition: 2015

Copyright © Publisher

Published by:
Satish Kumar Jain for CBS Publishers & Distributors Pvt. Ltd.,
4819/XI Prahlad Street, 24 Ansari Road, Daryaganj, New Delhi - 110002
delhi@cbspd.com, cbspubs@airtelmail.in • www.cbspd.com
Ph.: 23289259, 23266861, 23266867 • Fax: 011-23243014

Corporate Office: 204 FIE, Industrial Area, Patparganj, Delhi - 110 092
Ph: 49344934 • Fax: 011-49344935
E-mail: publishing@cbspd.com • publicity@cbspd.com

Branches:
- *Bengaluru:* 2975, 17th Cross, K.R. Road, Bansankari 2nd Stage, Bengaluru - 70 Ph: +91-80-26771678/79 • Fax: +91-80-26771680
  E-mail: cbsbng@gmail.com, bangalore@cbspd.com
- *Chennai:* No. 7, Subbaraya Street, Shenoy Nagar, Chennai - 600030
  Ph: +91-44-26681266, 26680620 • Fax: +91-44-42032115
  E-mail: chennai@cbspd.com
- *Kochi:* 36/14, Kalluvilakam, Lissie Hospital Road, Kochi - 682018
  Ph: +91-484-4059061-65 • Fax: +91-484-4059065
  E-mail: cochin@cbspd.com
- *Mumbai:* 83-C, Dr. E. Moses Road, Worli, Mumbai - 400018
  Ph: +91-9833017933, 022-24902340/41 • E-mail: mumbai@cbspd.com
- *Pune:* Bhuruk Prestige, Sr. No. 52/12/2+1+3/2,
  Narhe, Haveli (Near Katraj-Dehu Road Bypass), Pune - 411041
  Ph: +91-20-64704058/59, 32342277 • E-mail: pune@cbspd.com

Representatives:
- Hyderabad: 0-9885175004
- Nagpur: 0-9021734563
- Vijayawada: 0-9000660880
- Kolkata: 0-9831437309, 0-9051152362
- Patna: 0-9334159340

Printed at: Goyal Offset Printers

DIVINE INSPIRATION

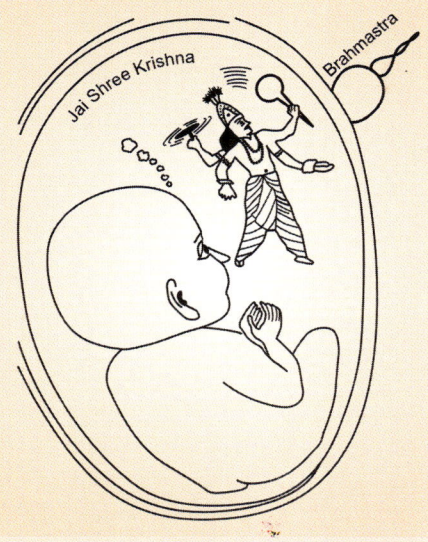

We equate **Paediatric Surgery** to **Bhagwan Krishna**. As Bhagwan Krishna saved life of Parikshit, son of Abhimanu in Uttara's womb (the lone survivor among Pandavas), similarly Paediatric Surgery (a branch of medicine) saves newborn with congenital malformations. Just like Bhagwan Krishna chose Vasudevji to cross the mighty river Yamuna, similarly, we really need a Godfather from Paediatric Surgery to carry forward the sinking superspecialty of Paediatric Surgery. In present era, when other so-called glamorous superspecialties like Plastic, Urology and Cardiac surgeries have overshadowed the rather "Untouchable branch" of Paediatric Surgery, we need a soul like Mahatma Gandhi to uplift the branch of Paediatric Surgery.

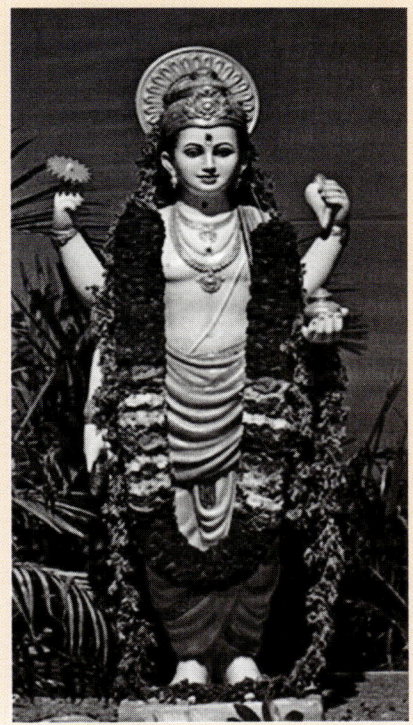

Dhanvantari
The GOD of Medicine

During Samudra Manthan, out of fourteen Ratnas who emerged from the ocean, one of them was Dhanvantari, "The God of Medicine". We are indebted to him for curing all ailments of the world. We pay our obeisance to Dhanvantari before embarking on the subject.

OUR TRIBUTE

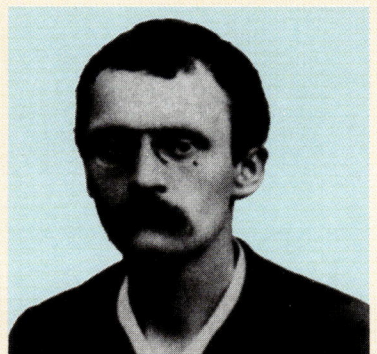

César Roux (1857-1934)

It would be unjust to begin without the mention of César Roux, a Swiss surgeon, who described the Roux-en-Y procedure in 1893. Roux's original French report on gastrointestinal surgery was published in Revue de Chirurgie. The Roux-en-Y technique of gastrointestinal anastomosis is an extremely priceless method used in drainage of the stomach, esophagus, and the pancreaticobiliary tree. It is a Y-shaped surgical anastomosis involving the small intestine. It is often used in restoring the continuity of the GI tract after resections for a number of diseases of biliary tract, pancreas, stomach and oesophagus. It would not have been possible for surgeons to perform and give results without the technique of Roux-en-Y. Over the last 100 years this technique has been utilized for restoring the gastrointestinal continuity. Even Roux had to bear condemnation for his wonderful technique in his endeavors. Also, the first successful surgical removal of a pheochromocytoma was performed by César Roux in 1926.

Reference: Hutchison RL, Hutchison AL. César Roux and His Original 1893 Paper. Obesity surgery, 2010; 20 (7): 953–6.

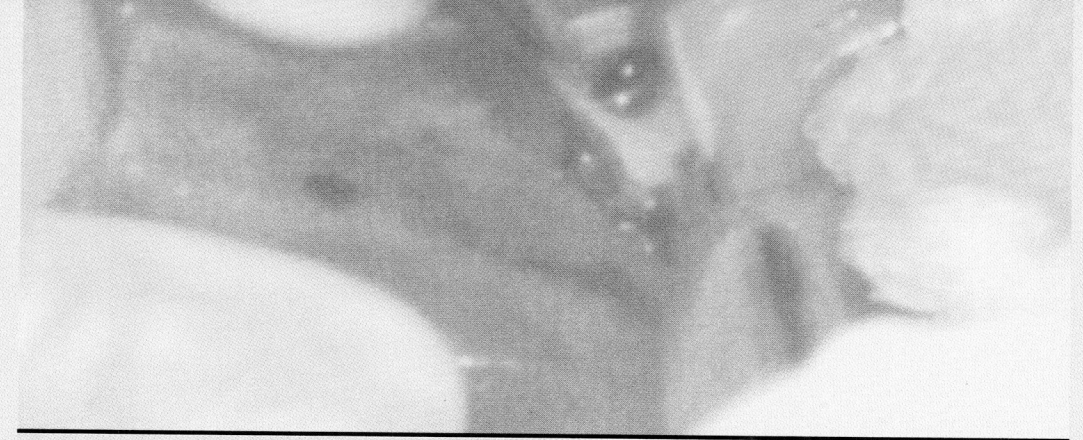

Preface

Choledochal cyst is an aneurysmal dilatation of the biliary tree presenting primarily in infants and young children. It is a potentially serious disease with a wide spectrum of presentation. A correct diagnosis and early surgical treatment is important because of the postoperative complications including malignant degeneration. Most of the scientific literature, particularly large paediatric case series regarding choledochal cyst, has been published by foreign authors, Japanese and Europeans. This prompted us to write this book. In this manuscript we are sharing our experiences with choledochal cyst, discuss its classification, aetiology, clinical presentation, complications, histopathology, surgical management and derive appropriate management recommendations in patients of choledochal cyst. Most of the cases were from the department of Paediatric Surgery, SPMCHI (Jaykaylon), SMS Medical College, Jaipur and the Department of Paediatric Surgery, NIMS University Medical College, Shobha Nagar, Jaipur.

We sincerely want to acknowledge Dr Ram Babu Goyal (Prof. and Head), Dr. L.D. Agrawal (Prof.), Dr. Arun Gupta (Prof.), Dr. Praveen Mathur (Prof.), Dr. A.K. Shukla (Prof.), Dr. Vineeta Chaturvedi (Prof.), Dr. Varsha Soni (Asstt. Prof.), Department of Paediatric Surgery, SMS Medical College, Jaipur; Dr. Alka Goyal, Department of Radiodiagnosis, and Faculty of Anaesthesia, SMS Medical College, Jaipur; Dr. Khyati Vaishnav (Asstt. Prof.), Department of Radiodiagnosis, and Dr Priyanka Golash (Asstt. Prof.), Department of Paediatrics, NIMS Jaipur, for helping us in our endeavour. We would also like to thank the faculty, residents and staff of the department of Paediatric Surgery, SPMCHI (Jaykaylon), SMS Medical College, Jaipur, and Faculty of Surgery, Faculty of Anaesthesia, and Faculty of Paediatrics NIMS University Medical College, Jaipur, for their constant motivation and help without which this endeavour would not have been possible.

Rahul Gupta
Shyam Bihari Sharma

ULTIMATE GOAL FOR A PAEDIATRIC SURGEON
"To bring smile on the face of children"

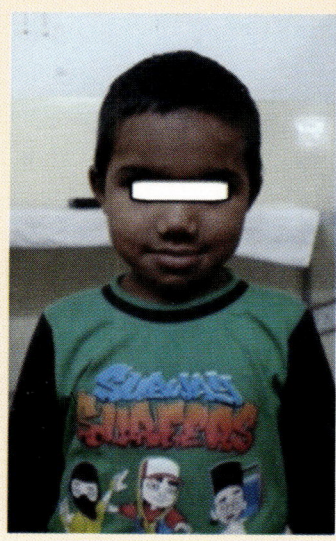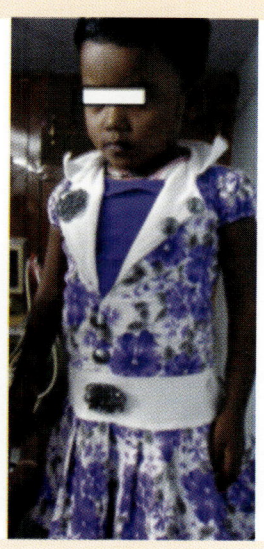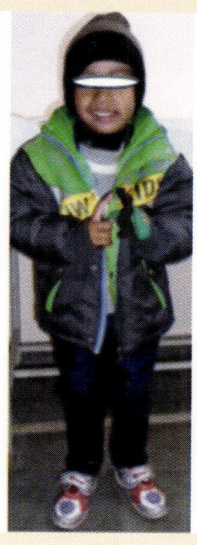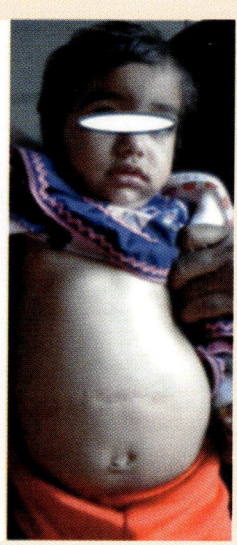

Efforts of surgical cure date back to the time of Maharishi Sushruta (1500 B.C.) known as "Father of Surgery" to Ambroise Paré, "Father of Modern Surgery". Dr. William E. Ladd is rightly called "Father of Pediatric Surgery" for his immense contribution to congenital anomalies of newborn. He was the first surgeon who committed himself entirely to paediatric surgery after 1927. Dr. Alfred Blalock and C. Everett Koop contributed to surgical management of congenital heart disease and endotracheal anesthesia of infants, respectively. Present day paediatric surgical outcome has been possible due to the contribution of many surgeons. They are responsible to bring smile on the face of children who are affected with various surgical conditions. In our society, when female foeticide is so rampant in all the strata, from poor communities to rich and influential, it is indeed unimaginable the plight of female child born with congenital malformations. These female children are the ones most unwanted in the society. We believe that paediatric surgical community should continue to strive for the healing and betterment of the children, especially female born with congenital malformations.

To me the ideal doctor would be a man endowed with profound knowledge of life and of the soul, intuitively divining any suffering or disorder of whatever kind, and restoring peace by his mere presence.

Henri Amiel

MESSAGE TO NEW GENERATION

We believe that stalwarts of Paediatric Surgery should persuade the budding doctors to choose this "Superspeciality" and encourage them to develop scientific temper. They should promote research in this field for prevention and enhanced treatment of congenital malformations, and imbibe in them wisdom to serve the "Non Verbal".

Medical students who want to dedicate themselves and work for the children (future generations), especially females with congenital malformations (the ones who can't express themselves and the subdued), Paediatric Surgery should be the first choice for them. Come and become a Paediatric Surgeon.

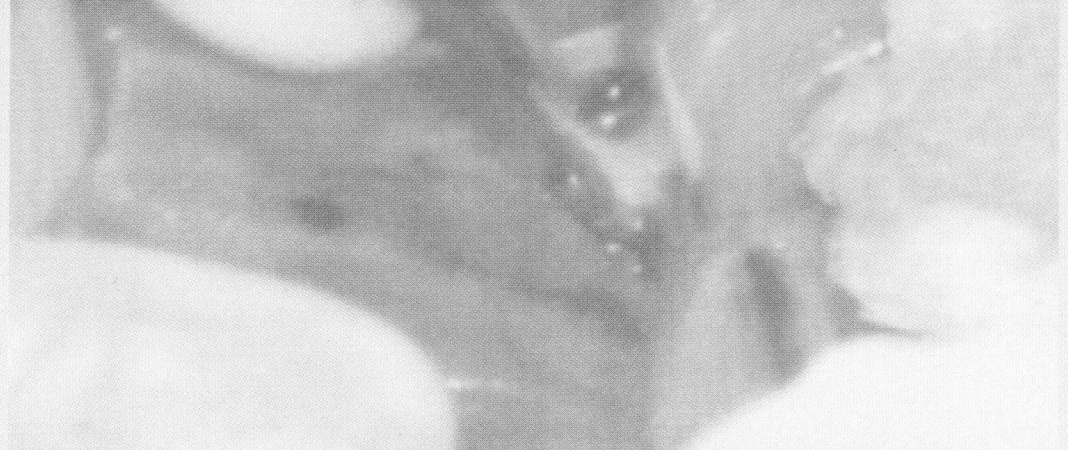

Contents

PEARLS

1. Five types of choledochal cysts are recognized as per Todani modified Alonso-Lej classification system (based on cholangiography).
2. Sixty percent cases present in the first decade of life.
3. Cyst-enterostomy (cystoduodenostomy or cystojejunostomy) are of historical importance.
4. Total excision with Roux-en-Y hepaticojejunostomy is the treatment of choice.
5. Lilly's procedure (Lilly's mucosectomy technique) is advocated for cyst densely adherent to the portal vein and adjacent vascular structures.
6. Type III cyst requires endoscopic management.
7. Type IVA disease (intrahepatic extension) rarely requires hepatic resection (selected cases).
8. Liver transplantation is indicated for Caroli's disease (Type V).
9. Type R (Roux-en-Y) – Cases requiring Roux-en-Y HJ are: Type IA, Type IB, Type IC, Type II, Type IVA & Type IVB of Todani's classification.
10. Type E (Endoscopic) – Cases requiring endoscopic management are Type III of Todani's classification.
11. Type V is entirely an intrahepatic disease and there is no extrahepatic dilatation of biliary tree as per the definition.

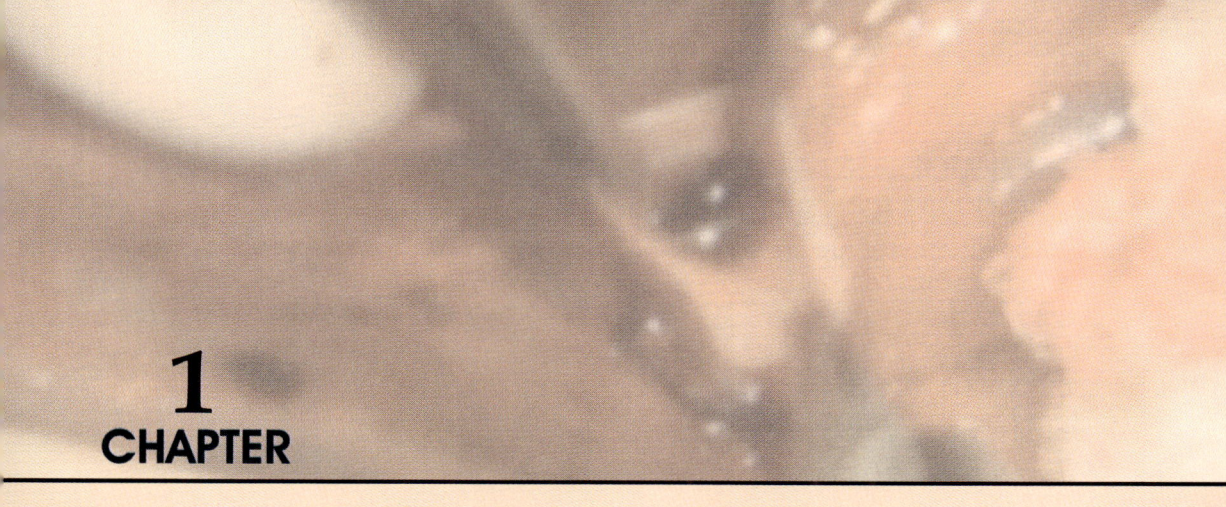

Incidence and Classification

INCIDENCE

Choledochal cyst is a rare congenital abnormality of the biliary tract and it accounts for approximately 1% of all benign biliary diseases[1]. It is defined as a aneurysmal dilatation of the biliary tree involving either extrahepatic or intrahepatic biliary ducts or both, occurring in approximately 1 in 100,000–150,000 live births in the western population[2, 3]. It is a biliary cystic disease and accounts for approximately 1% of all benign biliary diseases. As the condition is not only confined to the extrahepatic bile duct, the term "choledochal cyst" is in fact a misnomer and "biliary cyst" or "congenital bile duct dilatation" is probably more appropriate. Choledochal cyst is the traditional name. Incidence of choledochal cyst is 1 in 13,500 live births in the United States and 1 in 15,000 in Australia[3]. Most of the reported cases in the world come from East Asia and more than two-thirds of the cases in Asia are from Japan. It is common in Japan, with an incidence of 1 : 1000[4]. There is no evidence of increased incidence in the Hispanic population.

The **first reported** case of choledochal cyst was described by Vater & Ezler in 1723. It was then described by **Douglas** in 1852. In 1946 Shallon, Eger and Wagner reviewed the literature[5]. Initial classification by Alanso-Lej, Revor and Pessagno classified choledochal cysts into three main types, type I–III on the clinical and anatomic findings in 1959[6]. Type IV was first described in 1958. Alanso-Lej et al. classification was further updated by Todani et al. (based on analyses of cholangiograms) in 1977 who described five main types by adding type IV and V with several subtypes according to the location of biliary duct dilation[7]. Choledochal cysts have different forms of manifestation according to Todani's classification. Type I choledochal cyst can be subclassified into **Types Ia, Ib, and Ic**. This classification is most commonly used by surgeons[7–12].

TODANI MODIFICATION OF ALONSO-LEJ CLASSIFICATION SYSTEM

Todani modification of Alonso-Lej classification system of choledochal cysts is an anatomical classification (Fig. 1.1).

- **Type I** cyst, accounting for 95% of paediatric cases, is the most common. Type I is subdivided into type IA, type IB, and type IC.
  - **Type IA** is cystic dilatation of the common bile duct. There is marked dilatation of the extrahepatic biliary tree, partially or in its entirety. The gallbladder commonly arises from the choledochal cyst. The intrahepatic biliary tree is normal in appearance. Calculi may be visible within any portion of the biliary system.
  - **Type IB** is focal segmental common bile duct dilatation involving the most distal aspect of the CBD. A normal segment of common bile duct is usually present between the cyst and the cystic duct. The biliary tract proximal to the gallbladder is normal.
  - **Type IC** is fusiform choledochal dilatation involving the CBD and CHD. The dilatation may be up to several centimetres wide. The dilatation of type IC may be relatively subtle. The gallbladder arises directly from the dilated common duct. The intrahepatic biliary system is not dilated.
- **Type II** cysts account for about 2% of cases and consist of a true choledochal diverticulum. It may be as large as several centimetres in size.
- **Type III** (**choledochocele**) cyst forms 1.4–5.0% of total cases. It involves only the intra-duodenal portion of the duct. On T-tube cholangiogram, it is seen as a focal dilated segment of the intraduodenal portion of the CBD. The proximal biliary tract is normal in appearance. The choledochocele may be as small as 1–2 cm or, rarely, large enough to cause partial duodenal obstruction. It is analogous to the ureterocele. It is further subdivided into 5 types based on its relations to the ampulla of Vater and the pancreatic duct. In one subtype, type III may occur in intrapancreatic portion of the biliary tree. Because of chronic inflammation, openings of both CBD and main pancreatic duct (MPD) are stenotic, while opening of the **choledochocele into the duodenum is also narrow**. The presentation and management of all subtypes are identical. This sub-classification has not gained popularity among clinicians.
- **Type IV** cyst is subdivided into type IVA and type IVB.
  - **Type IVA** involves multiple intrahepatic and extrahepatic cysts, which account for 19% of cases in adults. It is rare in children. It shows gross cystic dilatation of both the CBD and CHD with extension of the cystic process into the intrahepatic biliary tree. The intrahepatic disease may present as multiple focal segmental dilatations, smooth fusiform ductal dilatation, on irregular nonuniform ductal dilatation. It is also described as cystic-cystic, cystic-fusiform or fusiform-fusiform to better delineate the nature of their intrahepatic and extrahepatic components.
  - In **type IVB** there are multiple cystic dilatations of extrahepatic system. It can have either a "string-of-beads" on a "bunch-of-grapes" (multiple diverticulae) appearance. The intrahepatic biliary tree is normal. It is very rare.
- **Type V** is dilatation of intrahepatic biliary tree. In other words, it is a congenital non-familial, multiple irregular dilatations of intrahepatic ducts (saccular or cystic) with stenotic segments in between.

Type V is also known as **communicating cavernous ectasia** or **Caroli's disease**. Caroli's disease is associated with congenital hepatic fibrosis and medullary sponge kidney. Simple Caroli's disease is isolated biliary dilation. Approximately two-thirds of patients with Caroli's disease also have extrahepatic disease. Repeated episodes of ascending cholangitis may result in stricture formation of CBD or the intrahepatic ducts between areas of saccular dilatation.

ANATOMICAL CLASSIFICATION
Todani modification of Alanso-Lej classification

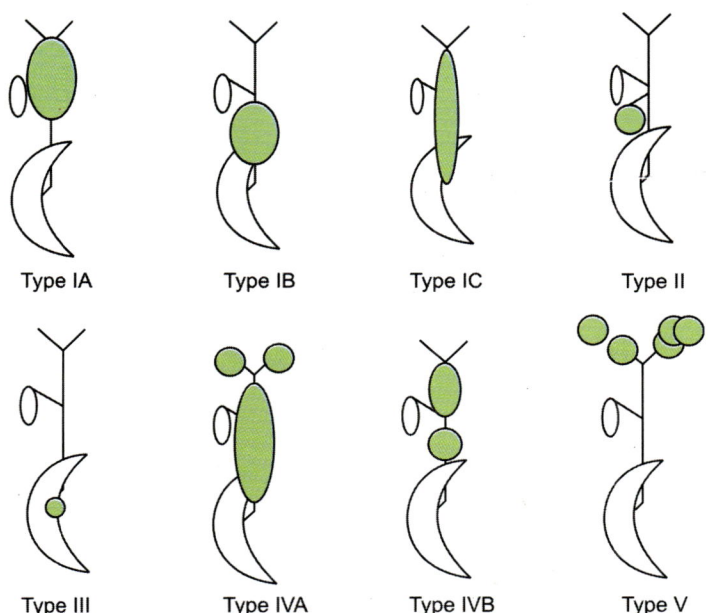

Fig. 1.1. Diagrammatic representation of Todani modified Alonso-Lej classification. Five types of choledochal cyst are presented, as evident by cholangiography.

Type I Dilatation of entire common hepatic duct (CHD) or common bile duct (CBD) or of segments of each. It is the most common type present in 95% of paediatric cases. It is further sub-classified into type IA, IB and IC.

    IA Cystic dilatation of either the entire extrahepatic bile duct or majority of it. It is like a saccule, into which the hepatic duct drains (Fig. 1.2).

    IB Focal segmental dilatation of the distal common bile duct, a very rare form.

    IC Fusiform dilatation of both common hepatic and common bile duct, without abrupt change of ductal caliber.

Type II Diverticulum from the common bile duct (Figs. 1.3 & 1.4) joined to it by a narrow stalk (very rare).

Type III Choledochocele, which is found in the intraduodenal portion of the common bile duct (5%).

Type IV **IVA** Multiple dilatations of the intrahepatic or extrahepatic biliary tree but most commonly, a large solitary cyst of the extrahepatic duct is accompanied by multiple cysts of the intrahepatic ducts. It is the second most common type, usually seen in adults (10%).

    IVB Multiple dilatations of the extrahepatic bile duct only.

Type V Dilatation of the intrahepatic biliary ridicules (Caroli's disease), left lobe usually affected (< 1%).

Todani classification does not include lesion type VI, which is an isolated cyst of the cystic duct, an extremely rare lesion. Unusual variants are also reported by authors, with isolated right hepatic choledochal cyst in a child, isolated left hepatic choledochal cyst in an adult. Type III and type IV sometimes coexist.

CLASSIFICATION BASED ON APBDJ

Japanese classify choledochal cyst into two groups, based on the presence and absence of APBDJ (Anomalous PancreaticoBiliary Ductal Junction) or PBMU (PancreaticoBiliary MalUnion), as they call it[10].

1. With APBDJ
   A. Cystic dilatation of the extrahepatic bile duct.
   B. Fusiform dilatation of the extrahepatic bile duct.
   C. Forme fruste choledochal cyst.
2. Without APBDJ
   D. Cystic diverticulum of the CBD.
   E. Choledochocele.
   F. Intrahepatic bile duct dilatation alone (Caroli's disease).

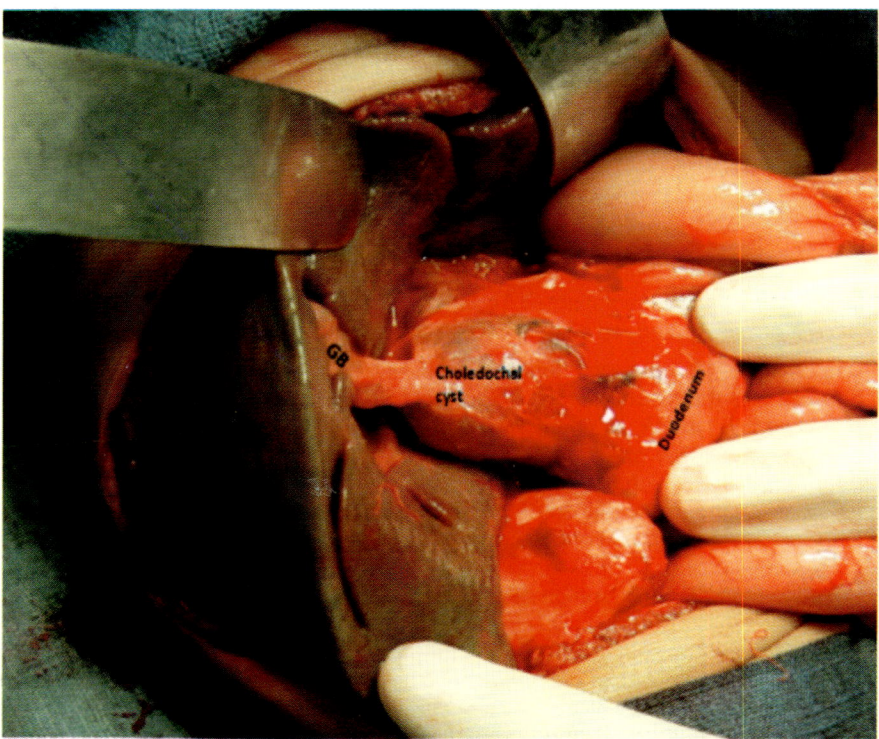

Fig. 1.2. Intraoperative photograph showing the classical variety of choledochal cyst (Type IA). Note: Cystic dilatation of the entire extrahepatic bile duct. The cyst is opening into the duodenum along with pericystic adhesions.

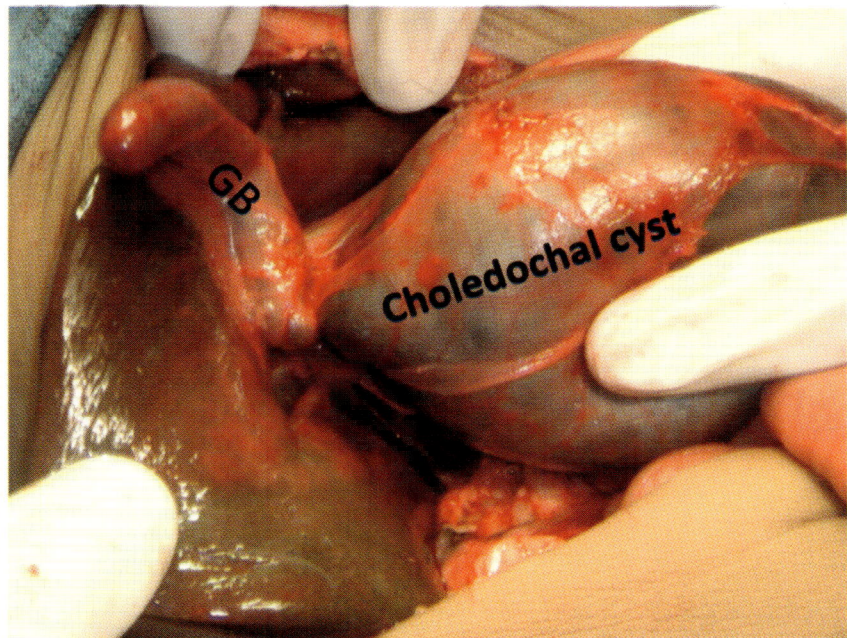

Fig. 1.3. Peroperative pictures of type II choledochal cyst. Gallbladder is seen along with the cyst.

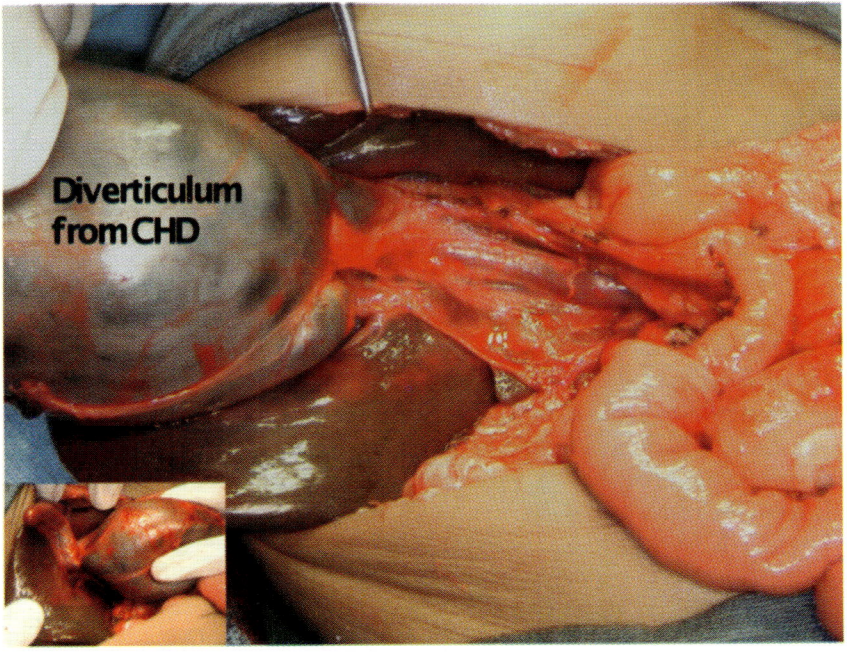

Fig. 1.4. Peroperative picture showing the cyst arising as a diverticulum from the CHD (Common hepatic duct), type II choledochal cyst.

Embryology and Aetiology

EMBRYOLOGY OF PANCREATICOBILIARY DUCTAL SYSTEM

During normal development of the human pancreaticobiliary ductal system, the ventral and dorsal pancreatic buds arise on opposite sides of the duodenum. Of the two pancreatic buds, ventral bud grows more rapidly than dorsal bud. Ultimately, ventral bud rotates to within the C loop of the duodenum and fuses with the dorsal bud. Dorsal bud forms the entire pancreas except for the head portion (uncinate process and inferior part of the head of pancreas), which is derived mainly from ventral bud. The duct system fuses in such a way that ventral duct and distal part of dorsal duct form the pancreatic duct, known as duct of Wirsung. The proximal part of the dorsal duct becomes the accessory pancreatic duct, known as duct of Santorini, which may or may not persist into adult life. The CBD and pancreatic duct normally unite within the sphincter of Oddi to form a common channel, termed the normal pancreaticobiliary duct, which opens into the middle portion of the duodenum. APBDJ (Anomalous PancreaticoBiliary Ductal Junction) and "long common channel" are responsible for pancreatic enzyme reflux and formation of choledochal cyst (Fig. 2.1).

AETIOLOGY

The aetiology of choledochal cyst remains speculative. However, the pathogenesis is **multifactorial** in origin[12].

The extrahepatic biliary system and ventral pancreas are formed between the fourth and the seventh week of intrauterine life. It commences in the Day 22 of IUL as a proliferating cord of cells from the endoderm of the foregut (at the site of future duodenum) at its junction with the yolk sac. It forms the endodermal portion of the liver and bile ducts. This cord (hepatic diverticulum) rapidly grows cephalad and ventrally into the septum transversum, and divides into 3 parts – the liver bud (large cranial part), the cystic diverticulum, the ventral pancreatic bud (small caudal part). The cells at the junction of these buds form CBD.

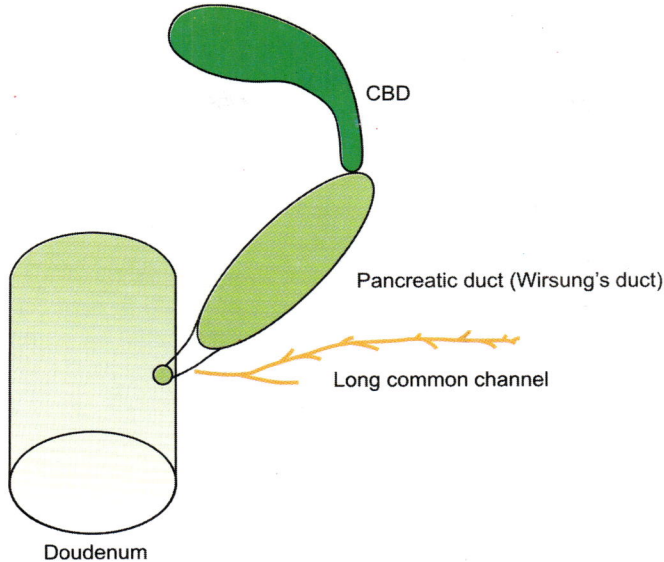

CBD

Pancreatic duct (Wirsung's duct)

Long common channel

Doudenum

Fig. 2.1. Diagram showing the long common channel and APBDJ as proposed by Babbitt in 1969. APBDJ and "long common channel" is seen, responsible for formation of choledochal cyst.

Dorsal pancreatic bud appears opposite the hepatic diverticulum at Day 26 of IUL[10]. This proliferation is followed by vacuolization, and coalescence of the ensuing lacunae results in formation of lumen. Choledochal cysts have been hypothesized to arise from inequality in the vacuolization of the biliary tract in early embryonic life (Yotsuyanagi 1936).

Choledochal cyst may be the result of an embryonic malformation causing "weakness" of the wall of the bile duct[13]. This weakness is coupled with a distal obstruction to produce the typical cystic anomaly[6]. This weakness of the wall has been termed "protodilatation status" and would progress to a choledochal cyst when the intraluminal pressure rises. Manometric studies have revealed that pressures as elevated as 50 cm H_2O are essential to force bile from the cyst into the duodenum – pressures sufficiently high to cause progressive dilatation of a cyst[6]. Antenatal ultrasound has documented the presence of choledochal cyst in utero, making it a congenital disease in nature.

The **Babbitt's theory** or **"long common channel theory"** (1969) remains the most popular and accepted. It holds true only for children and young adolescents[14]. This theory attributes the cyst formation to **Anomalous pancreaticobiliary duct junction (APBDJ)** i.e. abnormal connection between the pancreatic duct (Wirsung's duct) and the common bile duct. This theory was latter confirmed by Todani and co-workers in an analysis of ERCP and other cholangiographic imaging studies. For better understanding of APBDJ, let us understand the embryology of pancreaticobiliary ductal system.

The embryologic hypothesis of anomalous pancreaticobiliary ductal junction (APBDJ) relates the congenital aspect of choledochal cysts to **defective budding of the primitive pancreatic duct**. With the **outpouching of the ventral pancreatic bud from a more proximal position** (close to the liver) and when this faulty ventral bud rotates and becomes the pancreatic duct, a long common channel that drains both the biliary and pancreatic systems is created. This APBDJ is generally located far from the sphincter of Oddi (Fig. 2.1).

The normal length of the common channel is 0.2 to 1.0 cm (average, 0.5 cm), and the diameter is usually less than that of the normal pancreatic duct (3–5 mm in normal adults) because the common channel is encircled by sphincter muscle fibres. APBDJ precludes the formation of the normal flap valve which prevents pancreatic regurgitation into the common bile duct. There is a high rate of APBDJ in Japanese patients with choledochal cyst. Pancreatic bile duct junction is considered abnormal when the common duct on joining both bile and pancreatic ducts is > 15 mm or the junction is 6 mm outside the wall of the duodenum resulting in a long common channel. In other words, connection between the choledochus and pancreatic duct is outside of the duodenal wall. The length of common channel may vary from 10–45 mm. With distance > 15 mm, the junction is beyond the sphincter of Oddi and results in increased pressure allowing the reflux of pancreatic juice into the bile duct. The pancreatic duct pressure is 25 cm H_2O above CBD. In addition, in an experimental model, cylindrical dilatation of the common bile duct was induced by prolonged exposure to pancreatic juice. It is hypothesized that the **recurrent reflux of pancreatic enzymes into the choledochus** results in activation of pancreatic proenzymes causing inflammation, damage and weakness of bile duct wall. There are reported high trypsinogen and phospholipase A2 levels in bile of these patients, which enhances the inflammation and bile duct breakdown. Distal obstruction then leads to progressive dilation of the biliary tree and formation of choledochal cyst. This is supported by presence of amylase in a choledochal cyst[14]. Miyano & Yamataka have documented such abnormal junction in 90–100% of patients with choledochal cysts[15]. It is believed that distal obstruction combined with pancreaticobiliary reflux in utero is responsible for production of choledochal cyst. In children who present with recurrent pancreatitis and normal CBD, APBDJ should be suspected. Wong & Lister suggested that APBDJ is caused by arrested migration of pancreatobiliary junction into the duodenal wall before 8th week of gestation.

APBDJ may occur without choledochal dilatation, and this has been termed a **forme fruste choledochal cyst**[15]. In this entity patients present with typical symptoms of choledochal cyst, having associated APBDJ but without dilation of biliary ducts.

Also presence of a long common channel does not warrant development of a choledochal cyst. If we consider the relationship between APBDJ and the resultant dilatation of the CBD, Caroli disease is seen to be a distinct disease entity. Also, type II cyst seems to be a variation in anatomy rather than true dilatation of CBD.

Opponents of Babbitt's theory, in their experiments on animal models, created APBDJ and **induced fusiform dilatation of CBD** rather than cystic dilatation. Also patients with **forme fruste choledochal cyst** are exceptions. They also believe that role of pancreatic enzymes in the development of choledochal cyst has been overstated. The reasons being the functional immaturity of pancreatic enzymes in the early intrauterine life and at this time choledochal cysts have been diagnosed (15 weeks). This is true for the neonatal period also.

Recently, abnormal function (spasm/dysautonomia) of the sphincter of Oddi has been reported to predispose to pancreatic reflux into the biliary tree and choledochal cysts obstruction[16].

Congenital theory, with inadequate autonomic innervations, with abnormally few ganglion cells in the narrow portion of the common bile duct, resulting in a functional obstruction and proximal dilatation in the same manner as Hirschsprung's disease or achalasia of esophagus has been proposed[17]. **Type IVA cysts** are more common in adults than in children, raising the likelihood that lesions may be congenital, and they may progress with time.

Type II may represent the end stage of a healed prenatal rupture of common duct. **Type III** may just be **biliary duplication cysts**, while lining of choledochoceles can be duodenal or biliary epithelium, and some authors believe that these may be either duodenal or biliary duplication cysts[18]. Obstruction of ampulla of Vater may result in localized dilation of distal intramural bile duct resulting in **Type III cyst**.

Obstruction of the CBD is another etiological hypothesis for choledochal cysts and is also supported by other animal models (Spitz). In neonatal animal models, ligation of the common bile duct causes a dilatation morphologically resembling a **type I** choledochal cyst, while in adults, generalized dilatation of the whole biliary system is seen. Radiological and histological evaluation of paediatric patients clearly demonstrates that **stenosis in distal segment or APBDJ** is closely associated with cystic dilatation of CBD.

There are reports of **congenital web** at the lower end of the common bile duct in association with a type I choledochal cyst.

Distal ductal stenosis with abnormal insertion (ectopic distal) of duct into the duodenum, congenital stenosis of distal CBD, persistence of epithelial membrane and abnormality of valve are other proposed suggestions (Ito and co-workers). Intermittent obstruction from mucus plugs has been reported by Ando and associates.

In 1974, Landing hypothesized that neonatal hepatitis, biliary atresia, and choledochal cyst represented a spectrum of manifestations of what he called "infantile obstructive cholangiopathy". He proposed that the panductular sclerosis of EHBA and the extrahepatic distal obstruction responsible for the formation of the choledochal cyst were due to a perinatal infectious cholangitis (most likely of viral origin), which progressed to a fibrotic scarring of the biliary tract[19]. Viral infections, most likely reovirus which was detected in 3/4th of patients with choledochal cysts in one study, can explain acquired or adult-onset choledochal cyst[20]. Real-time polymerase chain reaction has demonstrated high levels of reoviral RNA in biliary tissues from patients with choledochal cysts compared with controls[20]. Possibility of viral infection of ganglion neurons causing oligoganglionosis and subsequent fibrosis of the lower end of the biliary tract has been proposed by one research.

Choledochal cyst in association with biliary atresia has been reported in infants. Also, choledochal cyst in association with congenital hepatic fibrosis has been seen. Familial cases point to a possible genetic factor predisposing to formation of choledochal cysts. There are reports of a mother and daughter, siblings and of dizygotic twins having choledochal cyst. Also, female predominance (sex-linked defect) and higher incidence in Japanese suggest a genetic etiology.

The cause of Caroli's disease is unknown but may be associated with autosomal recessive inheritance. The likely mechanism involves an *in vitro* event that results in derangement in normal embryonic remodelling of ducts and causes varying degrees of destructive inflammation and segmental dilation of intrahepatic bile ducts. Caroli's disease has been associated to various chromosomal abnormalities, including an unbalanced translocation between chromosomes 3 and 8. It is believed to be a distinct clinical entity. Caroli's disease can occur with both autosomal recessive and autosomal dominant polycystic kidney disease. A mutation in the PKD1 gene has been recognized in a family with Caroli's disease and dominant PKD, and 2 mutations were report in the PKHD1 gene in Caroli's disease with recessive PKD. A strong association between type V choledochal cyst and congenital hepatic fibrosis, and also presence of numerous associated biliary anomalies, such as absent or double gallbladder, congenital stenosis of the hepatic ducts, annular pancreas, and sclerosing cholangitis with choledochal cyst point towards multifactorial etiology[6].

3
CHAPTER

Clinical Presentation, Associated Anomalies, Complications & Pathology

CLINICAL PRESENTATION

Choledochal cyst has a bimodal age distribution. It is usually diagnosed in childhood, with 60% diagnosed before the age of 10 years, while only 25% are detected in adult life[9]. The age in reported cases ranges from newborn to 80 years. Also, increasing proportion of patients with this diagnosis is being seen in adults due to ever-increasing use of diagnostic armamentarium. They also have an unexplained female : male preponderance, commonly reported as 4 : 1 to 3 : 1. It is commonly reported as 1.5 : 1 in the paediatric population[11]. In our study, male preponderance was present, in contrast to the reported series in the literature[8]. We believe that the gender discrimination prevalent in our society and difference in rearing of the female child is the cause of under-reporting of the female cases in this part of the country[8]. Infants who have been diagnosed with a choledochal cyst prenatally do not ordinarily become jaundiced until 1 to 3 weeks after birth.

Choledochal cyst in childhood is frequently divided into an infantile group, and an adult group (classical paediatric group). Both forms differ in their clinical presentation and the pathological anatomy. Symptoms of choledochal cysts are characteristically intermittent but progressive.

Presentation is usually at the age of 1 to 3 months in the infantile group, with obstructive jaundice, acholic stools and hepatomegaly. Biliary obstruction is usually complete in these patients. This group consists of patients less than 6 months of age. Palpable mass in the right upper abdomen, with or without hepatomegaly is seen in late infancy[21–24]. Abdominal pain is not a feature in this group of children. Low grade fever may be present. Clinical picture is indistinguishable from that of biliary atresia. Characteristic features of cholangitis are not seen (Table 3.1).

In the so-called adult group of choledochal cyst, clinical manifestations generally become evident after the age of 2 years. The symptoms are: recurrent colicky pain in the epigastric region and right upper quadrant with radiation (often) to the right scapula followed by fever.

Table 3.1. Clinical presentation of choledochal cyst

	Infantile group < 3 months	Adult group > 2 years
Age at presentation		
Pain	—	Right upper abdomen dull pain
Jaundice	Obstructive variety (80%)	Acholic stools Intermittent
Abdominal examination	—	Palpable mass
Hepatomegaly	Hepatomegaly marked	May be present
Triad (Pain, Mass and Jaundice)	—	Present (17%)
Associated symptoms	Low grade fever	—
Complications	Biliary cirrhosis	Portal hypertension

This is due to intermittent biliary obstruction. In some patients mild form of jaundice is seen, which may be a pointer towards cholangitis. Other features are palpable right upper quadrant mass, and recurrent bouts of pancreatitis[21–24]. The classical triad of abdominal pain, jaundice and right hypochondrial mass first described by Alanso-Lej et al. is seen in this group (Table 3.1).

Jaundice is intermittent and obstructive in adult form, due to the formation of mucus plugs and biliary sludge. In case of long-standing jaundice associated with cholangitis, it may become hepatocellular.

Pain is usually vague in nature. It is difficult to express by non-verbal child. It is situated in the right hypochondriac region and radiates to the epigastrium, right iliac region, and back. Distension of the cyst may be the cause. The pattern of pain may be similar to recurrent pancreatitis, and is often supported by rise in amylase levels (which may be due to decreased amylase clearance or pancreatitis).

Mass is located in the right hypochondriac and epigastric region (right and above the umbilicus). It is soft/cystic, smooth, non-mobile, and may or may not move with respiration.

Table 3.2. Lumps which disappear and reappear

1. Choledochal cyst
2. Pseudocyst of pancreas
3. Hydronephrosis
4. Transient intussusception

The lump may sometimes disappear (Table 3.2).

Hepatomegaly may be seen in adult form, although it is less prominent than the infantile form.

Vomiting is due to distension of the cyst and compression effects.

Failure to thrive.

Choledochal cyst should always be considered in the differential diagnosis of obstructive jaundice or pancreatitis in children.

Patients with choledochoceles (type III) are not usually diagnosed until they are at least 5 years of age because the characteristic clinical symptom is abdominal pain of an intermittent nature that is non-specific[18]. Clinical presentation of Caroli's (type V) patients range from totally asymptomatic for many years to cholangitis, intrahepatic abscesses, hepatolithiasis, or jaundice[20–25].

The classic characteristic triad (Table 3.3) of abdominal pain, jaundice and right hypochondrial mass occurs mostly in childhood (0–17%) and approximately 7 times more frequently in children than in adults[21–24]. In our series, eight patients (14.5%) had the triad of choledochal cyst as shown in Fig. 3.1[8]. Eighty five % of children have at least 2 features of the triad at presentation, compared with only 25% of adults[25]. Abdominal pain is the most common symptom in adults, and may present with severe complications. If cholangitis continues for a long period of time, severe jaundice develops, and may result in septicaemia.

Table 3.3. Classical triad of choledochal cyst in 10% cases (0 to 17%)
1. Right upper quadrant pain
2. Jaundice
3. Palpable abdominal mass

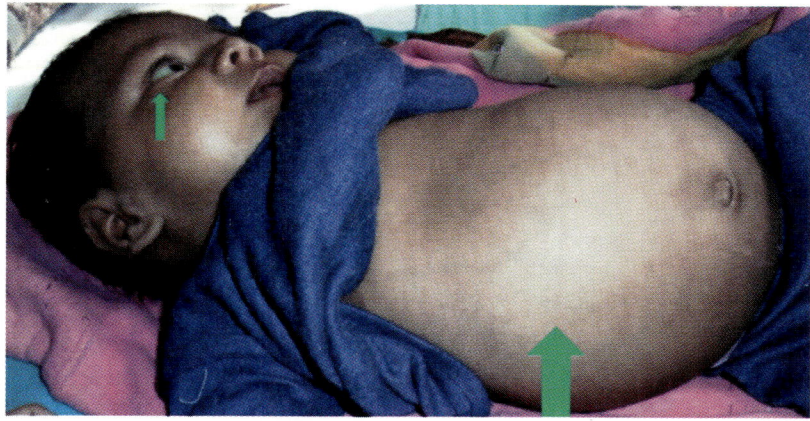

Fig. 3.1. One and half month female child of choledochal cyst presenting with jaundice (icterus as shown by small green arrow) and lump abdomen (as shown by large green arrow). The child had multiple crying spells with episodes of bilious vomiting.

Rare presentations include gastric outlet obstruction, neonatal bleeding tendency, duodenal intussusception, and portal hypertension.

In patients in whom the diagnosis is made in adulthood (gets unrecognized in paediatric age due to subtle and intermittent symptoms), biliary symptoms and cholelithiasis may be present. Recurrent cholangitis may be other presentation in adult counterparts. Diagnosis may be made at the time of laparoscopic cholecystectomy (for cholelithiasis) and after intraoperative cholangiography.

ASSOCIATED ANOMALIES

Associated anomalies include annular pancreas, duodenal atresia, malrotation, renal agenesis, polycystic kidneys, thoracic hemivertebrae[26].

COMPLICATIONS

Several complications are seen in choledochal cyst. The most common is recurrent episodes of **cholangitis**. It is related to complete or partial biliary obstruction. Complete obstruction may take place as a consequence of inflammatory stricture or choledocholithiasis due to protracted biliary stasis. **Pancreatitis** is a potentially serious complication, which is likely due to protein plugs accumulating in the Anomalous PancreaticoBiliary Duct Junction (APBDJ) leading to the activation of pancreatic enzymes by bile reflux[27]. 90% of the patients with choledochal cysts having a diameter equal to, or greater than, 5 cm developed pancreatitis as compared to only 9% of patients having cyst diameter less than 5 cm. The incidence of pancreatitis is higher in children as compared to adults. The incidence of pancreatitis has also been reported to be significantly higher in patients with a long (more than 21 mm) and wide common channel (greater than the size of pancreatic duct). Pancreatitis is associated with all types of choledochal cysts and is not related to either gender or race[27]. Pancreatitis is often a presenting feature in **type II cyst**. Patients with a choledochal cyst who present with recurrent acute pancreatitis may be cured with cyst excision alone.

In adult patients with choledochal cyst, chronic pancreatitis may result in dilatation of main pancreatic duct. Longitudinal pancreaticojejunostomy along with excision of the choledochal cyst and a Roux-en-Y hepaticojejunostomy may be mandatory. The same Roux limb is used for both the hepaticojejunostomy and the pancreaticojejunostomy.

Biliary obstruction is progressive due to recurrent inflammation and fibrosis, but may present **suddenly** due to common duct kinking as result of increased weight of the cyst. Direct compression of the portal vein is the mechanism responsible for the development of **portal hypertension** (PHT) in children. Extrahepatic biliary obstruction leading to **secondary biliary cirrhosis** (SBC) is the other cause of PHT. SBC has been found to occur in 10–50% of cases. The other causes include recurrent inflammation leading to portal vein thrombosis, and other unrelated aetiologies of cirrhosis. It is a rare complication associated with chole-dochal cyst, particularly in paediatric patients[27–30]. SBC leads to oesophageal varices and haematemesis. They are often associated with long-standing biliary obstruction and recurrent cholangitis. There is some evidence that even in patients with biliary cirrhosis and portal hypertension, disease regression is possible after surgical treatment[30].

Other common complications are **liver abscess**, **cholelithiasis**, **calculous cholecystitis**, **cystolithiasis**, **hepatolithiasis** and **portal aneurysm**[24, 28]. One of the rare complications of choledochal cyst is **biliary peritonitis** from **spontaneous cyst rupture**. It has been reported in 1.8–2.8% of patients in various series, while other claims it be 2–7%. Sometimes trauma may be the cause of cyst rupture in children. Spontaneous cyst rupture is most frequently seen in neonates and infants. Other cause reported is profound hypoproteinemia. Spontaneous perforation of the bile duct has also been associated with a multiple organ disorder, known as Ivemark syndrome, which consists of splenic abnormalities, cardiac pathology, and abnormalities of the gastrointestinal tract. It is extremely rare in adult counterparts. It has also been reported to occur spontaneously during pregnancy or labor.

The presence of protein plugs and the necrosis of the ruptured cyst wall would suggest that acute obstruction by protein plugs gives rise to obstructive jaundice, with subsequent rapid expansion of the cyst (associated with mural immaturity during infancy), followed by cholangitis with wall necrosis and eventual rupture. The site of rupture is often at the junction of cystic duct and CBD as this is a site of poor blood flow. It presents with acute abdomen. Peritoneal signs due to biliary peritonitis may be absent in some cases and preoperative diagnosis is usually difficult to establish. Signs pointing to spontaneous cyst rupture are bile containing ascitic fluid on abdominal paracentesis, hepatobiliary scintigram demonstrating an extrahepatic bile leakage and finally presence of bile-like peritoneal fluid at the time of emergency laparotomy. The perforation may be obvious immediately at laparotomy, or it may be concealed by an inflammatory mass/localized collection/spontaneous pseudocyst extending from the porta hepatis to the duodenum.

External bile drainage would be safer in emergency condition, especially when patients present late with sepsis and comorbidities. Peritoneal lavage and drainage through T-tube placed at the perforated site is carried out[27]. The distal duct is flushed with saline, greenish protein plugs are retrieved from the bile, after which cholangiography may be performed in such cases. We must be absolutely sure that distal duct is entirely clean prior to the abdominal closure. T-tube cholangiogram is then performed after about 4 weeks to study intra- and extrahepatic biliary tree, filling defects if any, and free flow into the duodenum. Reconstructive surgery is performed 6–12 weeks later. Reconstructive surgery may be tolerable even in emergency condition if a patient's preoperative condition is stable. Cyst excision with Roux-en-Y hepaticojejunostomy can be performed successfully in cases where adhesions at porta hepatis are not so extensive. Moreover, Lilly's approach appears to be very useful surgical technique in facilitating the primary excision of the cyst and thus preventing the morbidity associated with staged procedure, as per authors' experience.

Other complications of these cysts include liver abscess and occasional gallbladder perforation. Type III choledochal cysts can cause gastric outlet obstruction by obstructing the lumen or by intussusception, but is extremely rare. Despite substantial obstruction there is hardly any proximal biliary dilatation. Pancreatitis, cholangitis, history of previous biliary surgery and postoperative complications are more commonly seen in adults as compared to children.

Choledochal cyst is a premalignant state and the risk is high if untreated. Malignant change should be suspected in any choledochal cyst appearing after infancy, although in paediatric cases metaplasia and dysplasia are uncommon[31, 32]. It is mostly described in children and has been recorded in teenagers. Carcinomas of the biliary tract, including cholangiocarcinoma and carcinoma of the gallbladder are well-documented complications. Carcinoma in the head of pancreas in the region of APBDJ has been reported. The presence of cholangiocarcinoma in the cyst is reported in less than 1% of paediatric cases. The overall risk is 10–15%, and increases with age[33]. Most of the patients are in their thirties. The risk with an unresected choledochal cyst remains around 20–30%[34]. It usually develops in the posterior wall of the cyst. Risk of biliary tract malignancy is at least 20 times greater than that of the normal population.

Risk of cholangiocarcinoma in cysts is much higher in patients with APBDJ (32%) than in those without it (0%)[35]. APBDJ is categorized into two types: the pancreatico-choledochal (P-C) type, in which the main pancreatic duct enters the common bile duct, and the C-P type, where the CBD enters the main pancreatic duct. The incidence of C-P type junctions is higher in patients with carcinoma in choledochal cyst, while the incidence of P-C type ductal junctions is higher in patients with GB cancer. The number of bile duct cancer cases exceeds the number of cases of gallbladder cancer in the dilated bile duct with APBDJ.

Significant levels of carcinogens have been identified in the biliary contents in the presence of APBDJ. Pancreatic juice reflux secondary to APBDJ, chronic inflammation, bile stasis, possible development of carcinogens (conversion of bile salts to carcinogenic substances by chronic infections) and decrease of mucosal glands in the bile duct are the predisposing factors[35]. The **most frequent site** of carcinoma development is the cyst wall, although it may be at any height of the biliary tree[36]. Cancers are often first diagnosed at laparotomy, and can already be unresectable. Adenocarcinoma is the most common type and the usual site is extrahepatic bile duct[33]. Distribution of the types of cancer found in patients with choledochal cyst are adenocarcinoma (73–84%), anaplastic carcinoma (10%), undifferentiated cancer (5–7%), squamous cell carcinoma (5%) and other carcinoma (1.5%).

Chronic mucosal inflammation may result in **DNA damage** with subsequent mutations in oncogenes and tumour suppressor genes ultimately leading to cancer development. Increased expressions of Cox-2 (related to mucosal hyperplasia of gallbladder in APBDJ), increased telomerase activity, microsatellite instability and other molecular events have been suggested in causation of malignancy. Chronic post-obstructive infection by Gram-negative bacteria such as *Escherichia coli* metabolizes bile acids into carcinogens. K-ras mutations and overexpression of p53, which have been demonstrated in many other malignancies, are also present in malignant, precancerous dysplastic and chronically inflamed bile ducts in choledochal cyst and APBDJ. Inactivation of DPC4 gene occurs late in the progression of biliary tract adenocarcinoma.

PATHOLOGY

Pathological considerations in a patient with choledochal cyst are cyst, liver histology, gallbladder and presence of APBDJ. The cyst volume varies and it is frequently 400–500 ml. Also, volume above 13 litres has been reported. Stones in the cyst are decidedly uncommon. The bile is very thick and gallbladder is not dilated. The terminal common duct has normal histology. Type II cyst (diverticulum) is on a pedicle which may or may not have a patent lumen. The histological appearance of other forms of choledochal cysts is similar, with the exception of type III cyst.

Pathologic features (Figs. 3.2, 3.3 and 3.4) of wall of choledochal cyst are acute and chronic mucosal inflammation, mucosal dysplasia, disruption and relative absence of smooth muscle or elastic fibres. These findings are minimal in infants and gradually become more marked as patients get older. Inflammatory changes are usually most marked in intrahepatic component of type IVA cyst. Abnormal bile ducts may be present. Lining of cyst is devoid of columnar epithelium. Mucus-producing glands are infrequently seen along with microscopic bile ducts in the wall of cyst. Immunoreactive staining shows gastrin and somatostatin producing cells. Signs of inflammation and hyperplasia are primarily seen beyond 10 years of age and also in adults. There is frequently a huge amount of fibrosis of the cyst wall and remnants of mucosal lining are not seen in older age group. The cyst wall varies from 1 to 10 mm in thickness (thick-walled). Cyst wall is densely adherent to surrounding structures.

Microscopic evaluation of the type III cyst wall reveals duodenal mucosa rather than biliary epithelium in all paediatric patients, thus pointing a closer relationship to duodenal duplications. It is important to note that, although the outer lining of the cyst is always lined

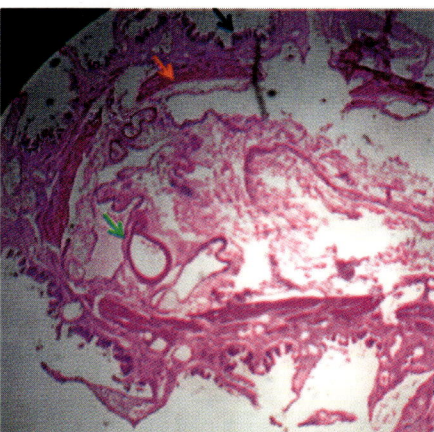

Fig. 3.2. Photomicrograph of choledochal cyst (hematoxylin and eosin ×4) shows a cystic lesion lined with mucous membrane (black arrow), underlying smooth muscle cell layer (red arrow), bile ducts (green arrow) and adventitial tissue.

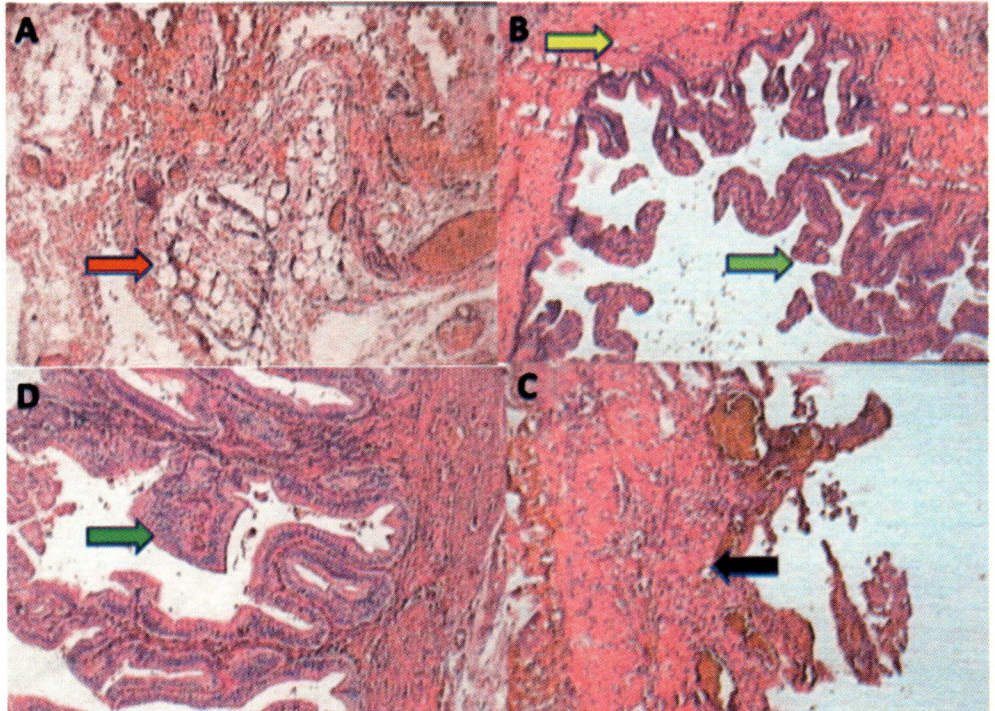

Fig. 3.3. Photomicrographs (hematoxylin and eosin) of choledochal cysts (A, B) shows loose fibrovascular lining of cyst (red arrow), fibrocollagenous tissue (yellow arrow), and biliary epithelium thrown into folds (green arrow). Microscopic examination (hematoxylin and eosin) of gallbladders (C, D) shows chronic cholecystitis (black arrow), normal mucosa and adenomatous proliferation (dark green arrow) with mild chronic nonspecific inflammatory cell infiltrate in the muscle layer.

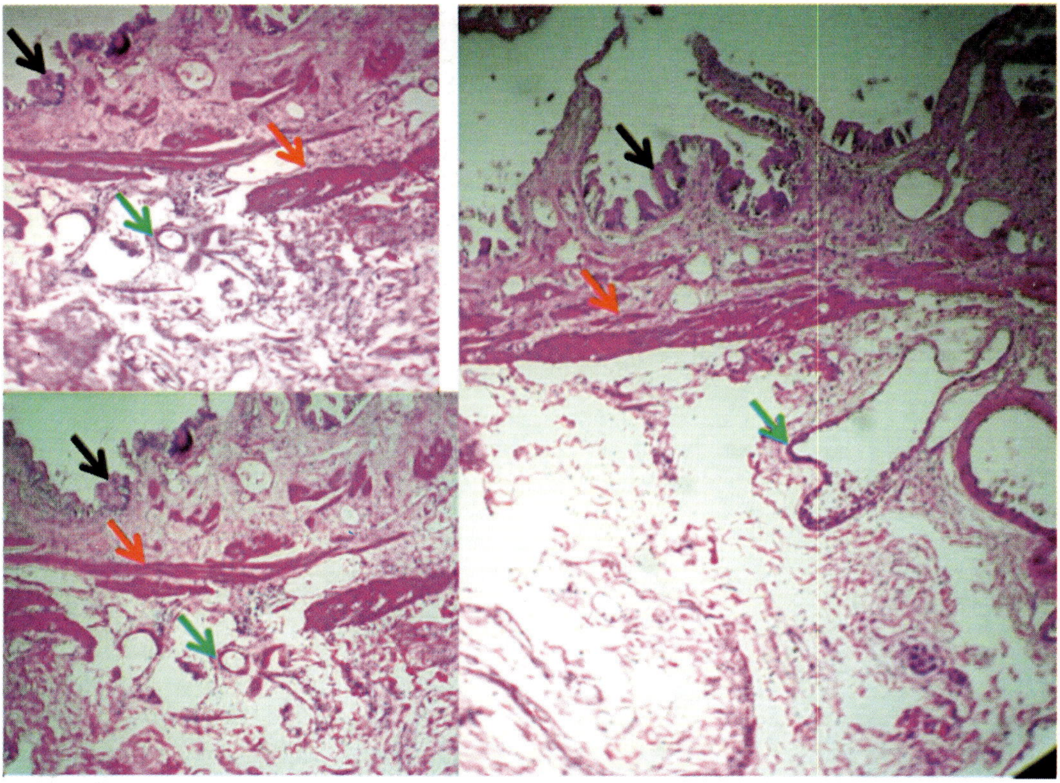

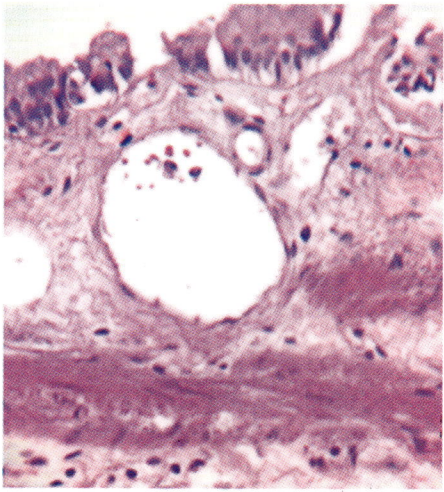

A

B

Fig. 3.4. A & B: Photomicrographs of choledochal cyst (hematoxylin and eosin ×10, and ×40 respectively) shows mucous membrane (black arrow) composed of single layer of columnar epithelium, smooth muscle cell layer (red arrow), underlying bile ducts, and adventitial tissue with mild chronic inflammation.

by duodenal mucosa, the inner lining can either be duodenal or biliary epithelium. The rest of the bile duct is usually normal on microscopic examination. Sludge or calculi may be present in the biliary tree. Only a handful of cases of adenocarcinoma associated with a choledochocele have been reported.

Findings of liver biopsy depend on the age of child *vis-à-vis* chronic biliary obstruction. It varies from normal to fibrotic or cirrhotic. Normal or mild bile duct proliferation is seen in newborn, while cirrhosis is in later age. Liver fibrosis may be seen at birth and is reversible with surgical repair. Liver fibrosis can be assessed based on Ohkuma's classification, grade 0, no fibrosis; grade 1, mild fibrosis confined to portal area; grade 2, moderate fibrosis with portal-portal area (P-P) bridging fibrosis; grade 3, severe expansive fibrosis with P-P bridging; and grade 4, liver cirrhosis with a reconstruction of hepatic lobules. The gallbladder findings in adult patients and particularly those with APBDJ include cholecystitis, cholesterolosis, adenomyosis, adenomas, polyps, and adenomyomatosis.

Differential Diagnosis, Investigations & Antenatal Diagnosis

DIFFERENTIAL DIAGNOSIS

Differential diagnoses are:

- Biliary atresia (Correctable biliary atresia)
- Congenital hepatic fibrosis
- Primary sclerosing cholangitis
- Congenital cirrhosis
- Pancreatic cystic lesions
- Pseudocyst(s)
- Impacted gallstone
- Cholangiocarcinoma
- Congenital biliary stricture (CBD)
- Cystic tumours
- Pancreatic disorders with bile duct obstruction
- Other causes of biliary tree dilatation.

PRENATAL DIFFERENTIAL DIAGNOSIS

- Simple hepatic cyst
- Biliary atresia
- Ovarian, omental, adrenal, renal or mesenteric cysts
- Duodenal or gallbladder duplications
- Dilated loops of the bowel
- Hydronephrotic renal pelvis
- Situs inversus.
- Giant cystic meconium peritonitis.

INVESTIGATIONS

Investigative tools are vital for the diagnosis of choledochal cyst in paediatric patients. They should be preferably non-invasive and effective because the children are averse to tests. Although, there is no specific blood investigation for choledochal cyst, CBC counts, liver function tests and coagulation profile are carried out for preoperative optimisation. The findings are consistent with mechanical obstruction of the pancreaticobiliary ductal system.

1. Conjugated hyperbilirubinemia (direct bilirubin).
2. Raised serum alkaline phosphatase: Elevated hepatocellular enzyme and alkaline phosphatase levels are nonspecific for choledochal cysts.
3. Elevated γ (gamma)-glutamyl transferase.
4. Raised amylase.
5. Deranged coagulation profile in long-standing biliary obstruction.
6. Leukocytosis with increased numbers of neutrophils and immature neutrophil forms may be noted in cholangitis.
7. Raised serum amylase and lipase indicates pancreatitis, but can also be elevated in the presence of biliary obstruction and cholangitis.
8. Serum chemistry levels may be abnormal if patient is vomiting (hypochloremic, hypokalemic metabolic alkalosis).
9. Increased CA 19-9 should raise the suspicion of malignancy in adults (in contrast to paediatric patient).

Paediatric patients with severe or intermittent abdominal pain ought to have a plasma amylase level performed. High levels associated with choledochal cyst are either due to clinically severe pancreatitis or partly may be due to diffusion of amylase through the denuded epithelium of the cyst wall in those with a APBDJ and high biliary amylase level which is described as 'biochemical' pancreatitis.

A soft tissue radiotranslucent shadow is seen on **radiogram or barium studies**. It usually displaces the right upper quadrant structures downwards, forwards, and to the left. Widening of "C" loop of duodenum is seen in barium study. Upper gastrointestinal series may show a filling defect due to bulge into duodenal lumen in type III cyst.

Ultrasound is an excellent first-line investigation with specificity of 97% in children[11, 37]. High resolution abdominal ultrasound is an excellent screening test. A dilated cystic lesion which communicates with the bile duct, separate from the gallbladder is seen on ultrasound (Fig. 4.1). It evaluates the entire intrahepatic and extrahepatic biliary system (Figs. 4.2 & 4.3)[11, 37]. Important considerations are size, contour, and position of the cyst, extent of intrahepatic duct dilatation, vascular anatomy, presence of pancreatic duct dilatation, intrahepatic/biliary tree lithiasis, signs of portal hypertension, splenomegaly and status of liver (fibrosis) or hepatic echotexture.

Treat the patient, not the X-ray.
James M. Hunter

The typical appearance of a choledochal cyst that is extrahepatic in location is that of an **anechoic mass in the region of the porta hepatis** that is clearly distinct from the gallbladder. In type III cyst, bile duct dilatation may be the only finding, due to its intraduodenal location and close proximity to the pancreas. Biliary ductal dilatation is also seen in choledocholithiasis, inflammatory stricture, periampullary carcinoma and other neoplasms in the head of pancreas. The common bile duct diameter measures less than 3–5 mm in healthy children and less than 2 mm in infants. In Caroli's disease or in type IVA cysts, multiple intrahepatic anechoic areas are seen. The typical feature of Caroli's disease is **string of beads** appearance with normal APBDJ and extrahepatic biliary tree on ultrasonography.

The limitations of ultrasound are evaluation of pancreaticobiliary junction and distal common bile duct due to overlying bowel gas. Also in case of large extrahepatic cyst, it is difficult to demonstrate continuity with the bile tract, which often is poorly defined with ultrasound due to overlying bowel gas.

Doppler ultrasonography discriminates cystic biliary structures from vascular structures. Portal vein thrombosis in patients with a history of recurrent cholangitis, cyst may be densely adherent to the portal vein and can be diagnosed with it.

CT scan is highly accurate investigation for confirming the diagnosis and offers a great deal of information that is helpful in surgical planning. It demonstrates a dilated cystic mass with clearly defined walls that is separate from the gallbladder and arising from extrahepatic bile duct (Fig. 4.4). CT scan endows better visualization of the distal CBD and head of the pancreas. Choledochal cyst is usually clear from its location and its relationships to surrounding structures (Figs. 4.5, 4.6, 4.7, 4.8 & 4.9). Extrahepatic cysts appear as low-attenuation areas in the region of the porta hepatis, while multiple low-density liver lesions, in place of focally dilated biliary tract are seen in type IVA (Figs. 4.10, 4.11 & 4.12).

MRCP is considered "gold standard" in the imaging of choledochal cyst and accurately defining the entire pancreatobiliary system, especially APBDJ[38]. It gives best projection image for showing the extent of the cyst as well as the best choice of surgical planning (Figs. 4.13, 4.14, 4.15, 4.16, 4.17, 4.18 & 4.19). It is non-invasive complete diagnostic modality. Its use may obviate the necessity of performing intraoperative cholangiography. MRCP was first named by Takehara in 1994. It is based on heavily T2-weighted pulse sequences.

Dynamic secretin-stimulated MRCP studies have been performed to understand the pathophysiologic characteristics of choledochal cyst. Non-breath-hold MRCP is the choice of imaging techniques in children with choledochal cysts. It is non-invasive, and does not involve ionizing radiation and potentially toxic contrast agents.

MRCP gives information equal to that of ERCP. It is also superior to CT, but in our resource-limited set-up, where facilities for sedating and carrying out the investigation in smaller children compounded with the non-availability of trained anaesthetist, makes it an extremely difficult endeavour. It is also expensive. We consider CT with contrast as investigation of choice in smaller children[8].

Radionucleotide scintigraphy (HIDA/DISIDA scan) is an investigation of choice for neonatal jaundice. It is safe in newborn. Scintigraphy follows the progression of an isotope from the biliary tract into the small intestine, and is reported to distinguish with 100% accuracy between choledochal cysts and biliary atresia[39]. In early 1970s, iodine-131 Rose

Bengal was used. Now scans are performed using technetium-99m imino diacetic acid derivatives, including N-(2,6-diethylphenylcarbamoylmethyl) iminodiacetic acid (DEIDA), N-(2,6-dimethylphenylcarbamoylmethyl) iminodiacetic acid (HIDA), p-isopropylacetanilido iminodiacetic acid (PIPIDA), and diisopropylphenylcarbamoylmethyl iminodiacetic acid (DISIDA).

Of all the IDA-derivative scans available, the DISIDA agent is lipophilic and less bound to bilirubin than other forms of the isotope. Scintigraphy demonstrates continuity of cystic structures with the biliary system, information about the drainage, obstruction and hepatic function. It is safe, atraumatic, and has been used for a long time in the diagnosis of choledochal cysts. The procedure involves intravenous administration of 74 to 185 MBq (2–5 mCi) of DISIDA after 3–4 hours of fasting, followed by imaging after injection with flow. Flow and/or blood-pool images are analyzed for the presence of a photopenic region corresponding to the choledochal cyst.

The role of scintigraphy assumes importance in order to diagnose bile leak following cyst rupture or after definitive surgery.

Percutaneous transhepatic cholangiography provides detailed imaging of the choledochal cyst, the noninvolved portion of the extrahepatic biliary tree, and the intrahepatic biliary tree. It involves transcutaneous aspiration and injection of contrast medium into the transhepatic route. It is associated with a high risk of bile leakage. It is reserved for older individuals with suspected choledochal cyst with dilated IHBR and severe jaundice or those with intrahepatic biliary cysts.

Endoscopic Retrograde Cholangiopancreatography (ERCP) is one of the most commonly used methods for diagnosis of choledochal cysts, especially in the initial management of biliary malignancies. It is performed by modern paediatric duodenoscope. It clearly shows the anatomy of the pancreaticobiliary junction. Endoscopy and ERCP demonstrate bulging and also dilated intramural CBD. Diagnosis of **APBDJ** is confirmed by this technique.

ERCP is the choice of imaging modality in choledochoceles (**type III cyst**) as it facilitates a therapeutic papillotomy simultaneously in these cases. Type III cysts assume a "cobrahead" appearance, as seen in case of a ureterocele. In addition, the typical extramural union between the pancreatic and biliary ducts seen with type I choledochal cysts is not a feature of choledochoceles.

ERCP is routinely performed in Japanese centers for the diagnosis of choledochal cyst and other biliary pathologies. ERCP is performed by retrograde injection of contrast and there is a high possibility of ascending cholangitis. It is an invasive technique and has potential complications like acute pancreatitis and there is a lack of cooperation from paediatric patients. It is unsuitable for repetitive use. We believe that, it should be reserved for adult patients. Also, MRCP has been shown to be just as good as ERCP as far as the diagnosis of choledochal cyst is concerned[38].

Angiography is performed when major vascular complications like hepatic artery aneurysms are associated with choledochal cyst.

A smart mother makes often a better diagnosis than a poor doctor.
August

It is difficult to distinguish choledochal cysts from biliary atresia with biliary cysts even after good preoperative work-up. A survey of the American Academy of Pediatrics – Surgery Section found that 13% of patients with cystic dilation of the CBD had biliary atresia. Choledochal cysts are larger than biliary cysts associated with biliary atresia in reported cases. It has been recommended that when the diameter of the CBD is greater than 1 cm, then there is a greater probability of encountering choledochal cyst.

The assessment and difference between important investigations have been summarized in Table 4.1.

Table 4.1. The assessment between different investigation modalities

Variables	DISIDA scan	MRCP	ERCP
1. Invasive procedure (endoscopy)	No	No	Yes
2. Expertise of the operator (pediatric gastroenterologist/radiologist)	Low	Low	High
3. Lack of cooperation from pediatric patients	No	Yes, usually with small children	Yes
4. General anaesthesia	No	Sedation/general anaesthesia	General anaesthesia
5. Radiological contrast agent	Yes	Yes	Yes
6. Radiation exposure	Yes	No	Yes
7. 3D reconstruction	Yes	No	No
8. Identification of APBDJ	+/–	+/– Partially replace ERCP	Brilliant
9. Visualisation of pancreatic duct proximal to obstruction	No	Yes	No
10. Relationship to adjoining structures	No	Brilliant	No
11. Possibility of ascending cholangitis	No	No	Present
12. Limitations	—	Patient's age, size, and weight	Paediatric duodenoscope

ANTENATAL DIAGNOSIS

Antenatal diagnoses can be made on serial high-resolution maternal ultrasound. An increasing number of type IA cysts are detected by antenatal ultrasound. It may be diagnosed as early as 15 to 25 weeks of gestation. Diagnosis in 37 weeks (late third trimester) has been made. It is a screening test, and is not necessarily reliable. It is extremely difficult to distinguish it from other biliary cysts. It may differentiate it from biliary atresia according to relative rates of enlargement of the duct diameter[37]. It is agreed that whenever choledochal cyst is suspected postnatal ultrasound is mandatory.

Diagnosis is not the end, but the beginning of practice.
Martin H. Fischer

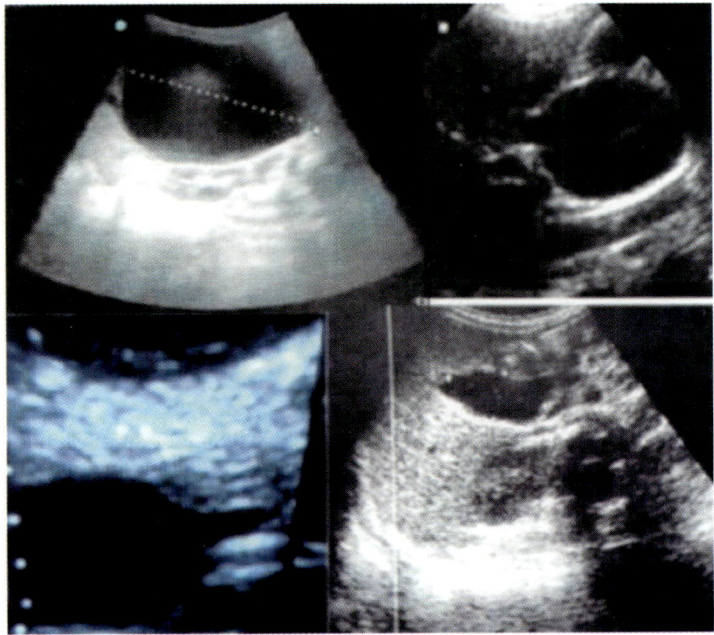

Fig. 4.1. Ultrasound images showing well-defined anechoic cystic lesion involving the extrahepatic biliary tree characteristic of choledochal cyst.

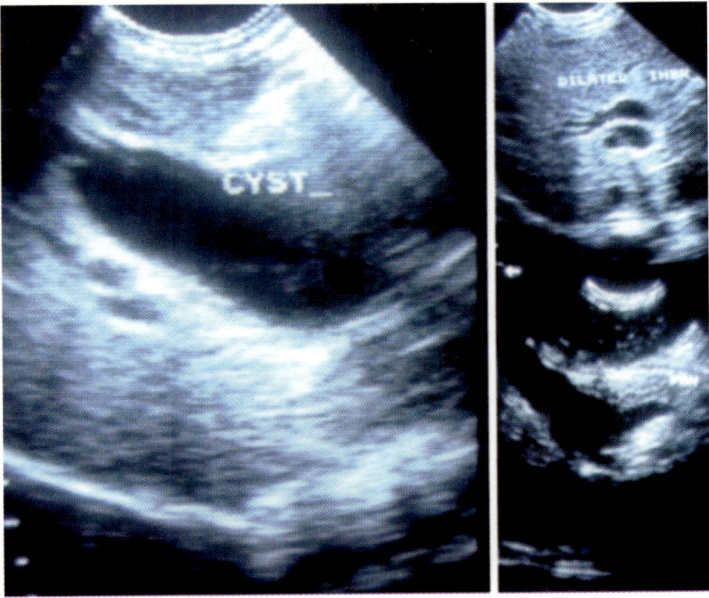

Fig. 4.2. Ultrasound images showing well-defined anechoic cystic lesion involving the extrahepatic biliary tree (choledochal cyst) and dilatation of IHBR (intrahepatic biliary radicles) characteristic of choledochal cyst type IA.

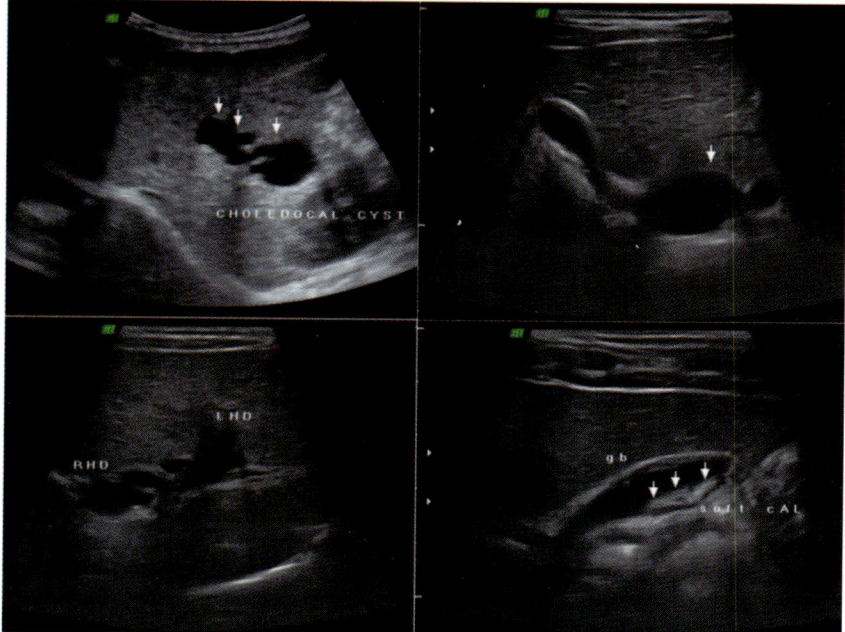

Fig. 4.3. Ultrasound image showing well-defined anechoic cystic lesion involving the extrahepatic biliary tree with intrahepatic dilatation of LHD (Left Hepatic Duct) and RHD (Right Hepatic Duct) characteristic of type IVA choledochal cyst. A soft calculus is seen in the gallbladder (shown by arrows).

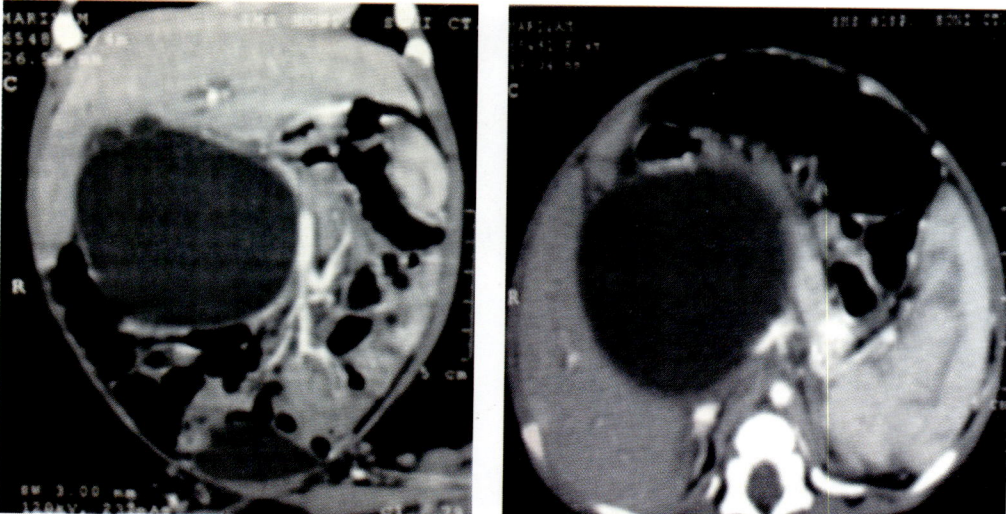

Fig. 4.4. CECT scan (coronal sections) images showing well-defined non-enhancing cystic lesion involving the extrahepatic biliary tree characteristic of type IA choledochal cyst. The cyst is typically filled with bile, which produces water-like attenuation. Enhancing pancreatic parenchyma is seen on medial aspect of the cyst.

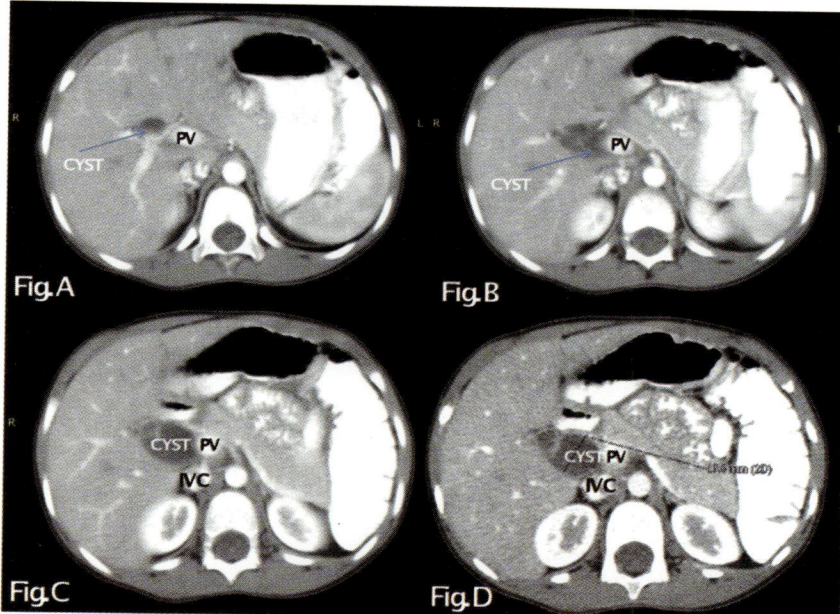

Fig. 4.5. CECT images showing well-defined non-enhancing cystic lesion involving the extrahepatic biliary tree characteristic of type IA choledochal cyst. The images are marked A to D (craniocaudally). Cyst: Blue arrow; Portal vein: PV, IVC: Inferior vena cava. Proximal extension of dilated CHD is seen in Fig. A. Close relationship of choledochal cyst to portal vein is seen. On exploration, it was found to be densely stuck to portal vein, which necessitated a Lilly's procedure.

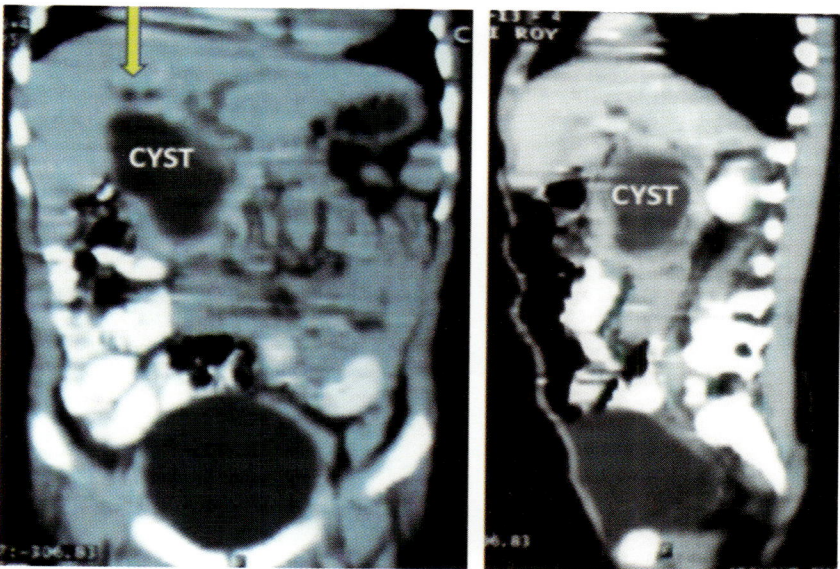

Fig. 4.6. CECT images (coronal sections) reveal findings characteristic of choledochal cyst. Yellow arrow: IHBR.

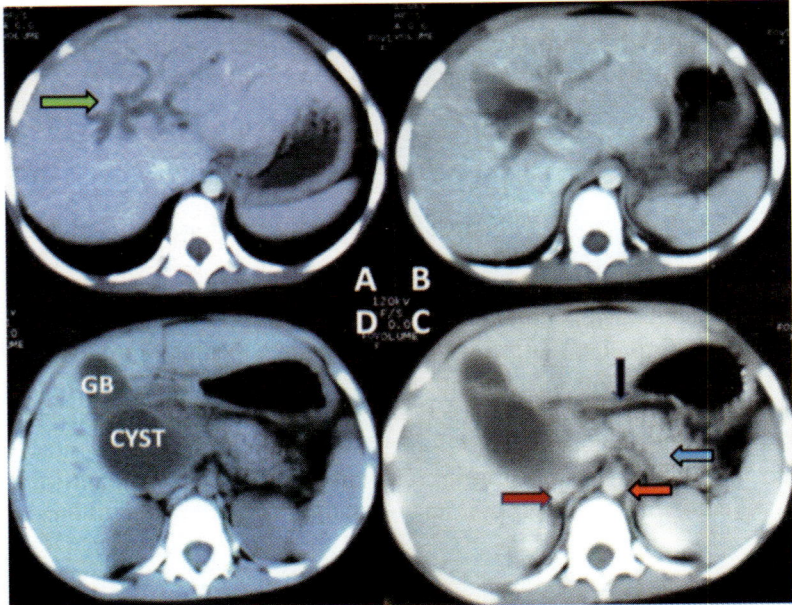

Fig. 4.7. CT images reveal well-defined non-enhancing cystic lesion involving the extrahepatic biliary tree characteristic of type IA choledochal cyst along with dilatation of IHBR (green arrow). The images are marked A to D (craniocaudally). Red arrow: Descending aorta, Maroon arrow: IVC (Inferior vena cava), Black arrow: Bowel gas, Blue arrow: Pancreatic parenchyma.

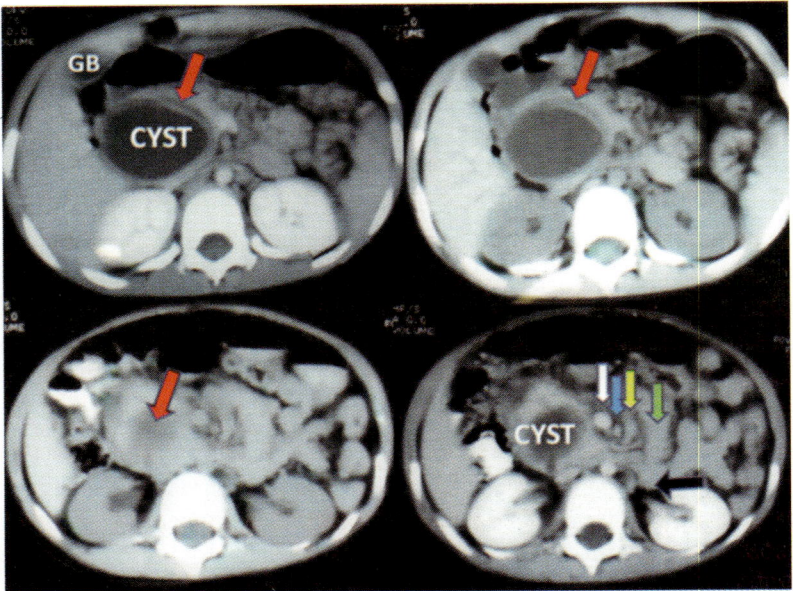

Fig. 4.8. CT images reveal well-defined non-enhancing cystic lesion (red arrow) characteristic of choledochal cyst. White arrow: SMV, blue arrow: SMA, yellow & green arrow: Bowel loops.

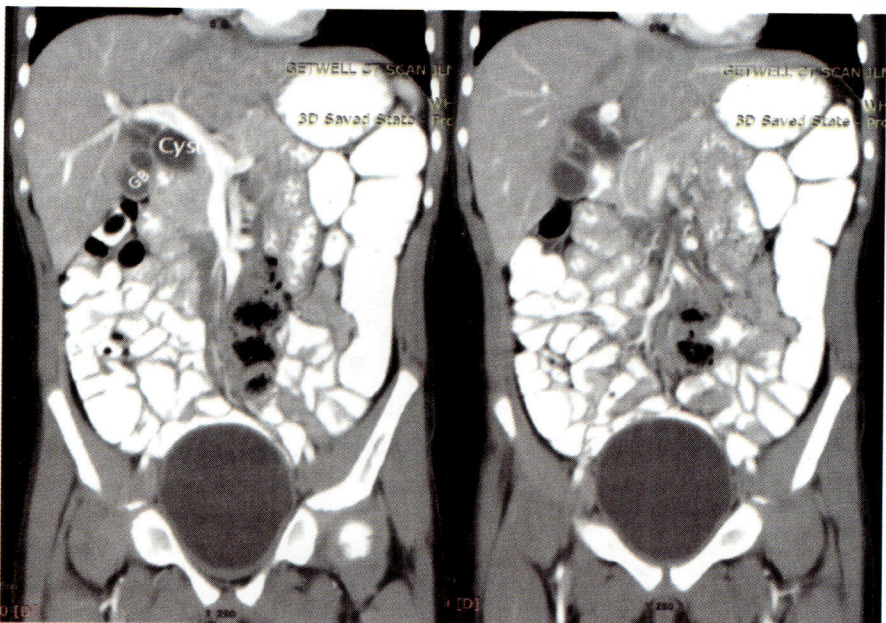

Fig. 4.9. CECT images (coronal sections) showing proximal extent of type IA choledochal cyst.

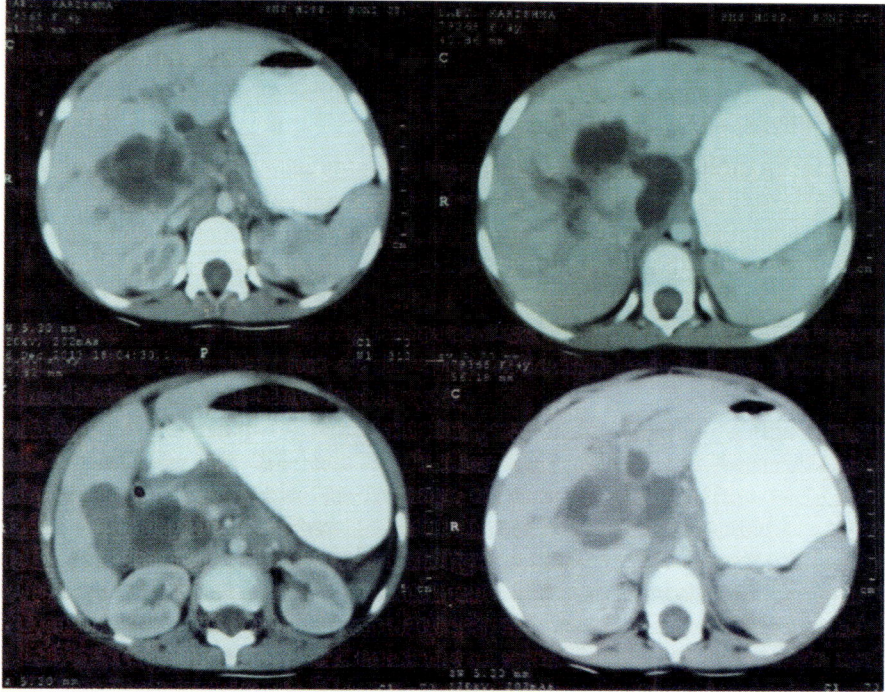

Fig. 4.10. CECT images (transverse sections) showing type IVA choledochal cyst.

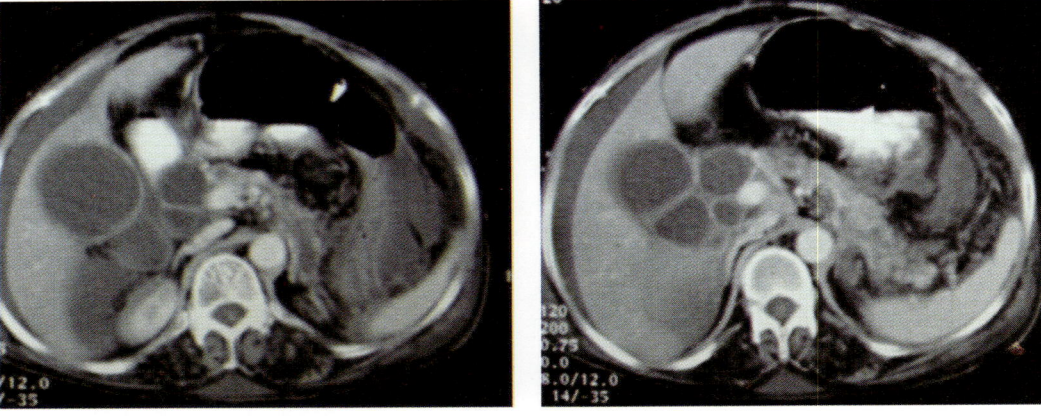

Fig. 4.11. CECT images showing cystic dilatation of both extra- and intrahepatic dilatation of biliary tree characteristic of type IVA choledochal cyst.

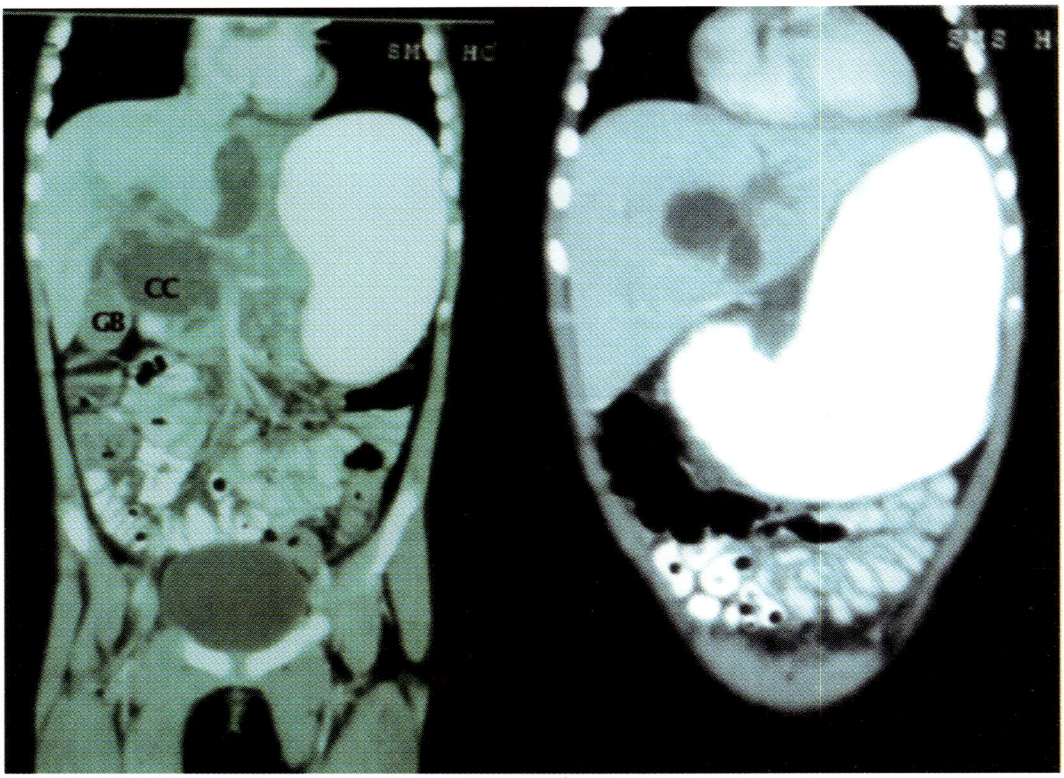

Fig. 4.12. CECT images (coronal sections) showing type IVA choledochal cyst.

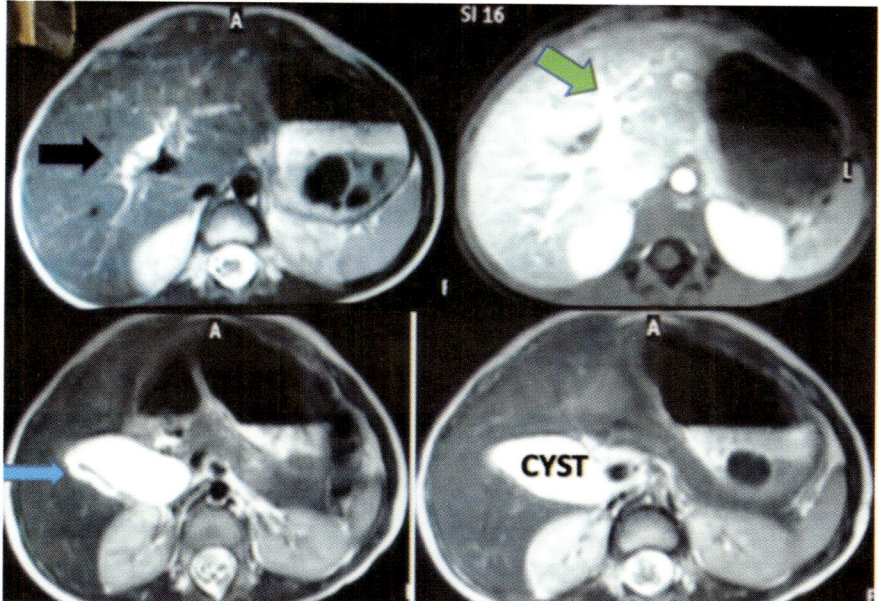

Fig. 4.13. MRCP images (T2 signal) showing type IA choledochal cyst with dilated IHBR (black and green arrows) as shown in upper images, close relationships with duodenum and vascular structures is shown in lower images. Also long cystic duct is shown by blue arrow.

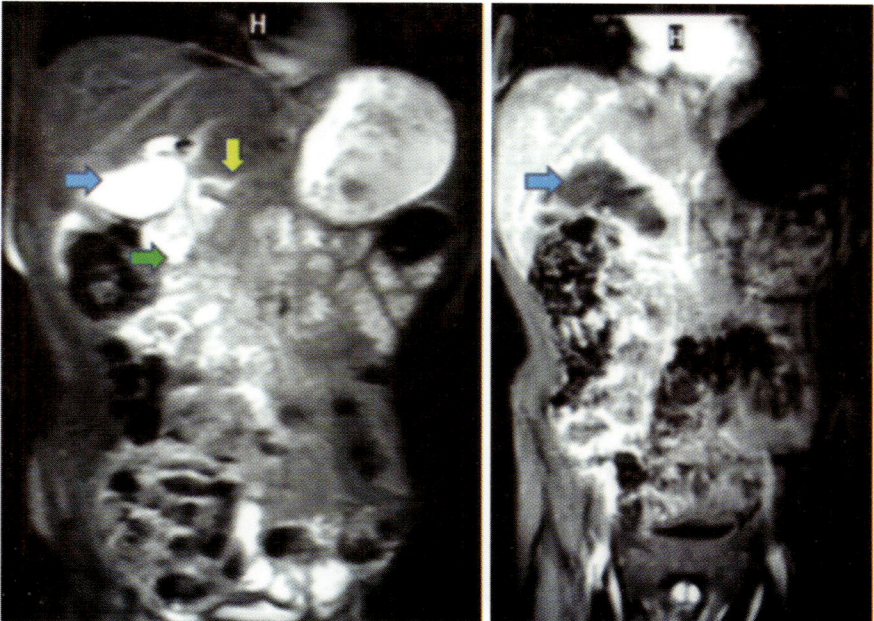

Fig. 4.14. MRI images (coronal sections) with T2 signal on left and T1 signal on right, showing type IA cyst (green arrows). IHBR is shown by yellow arrow and gallbladder by green arrow.

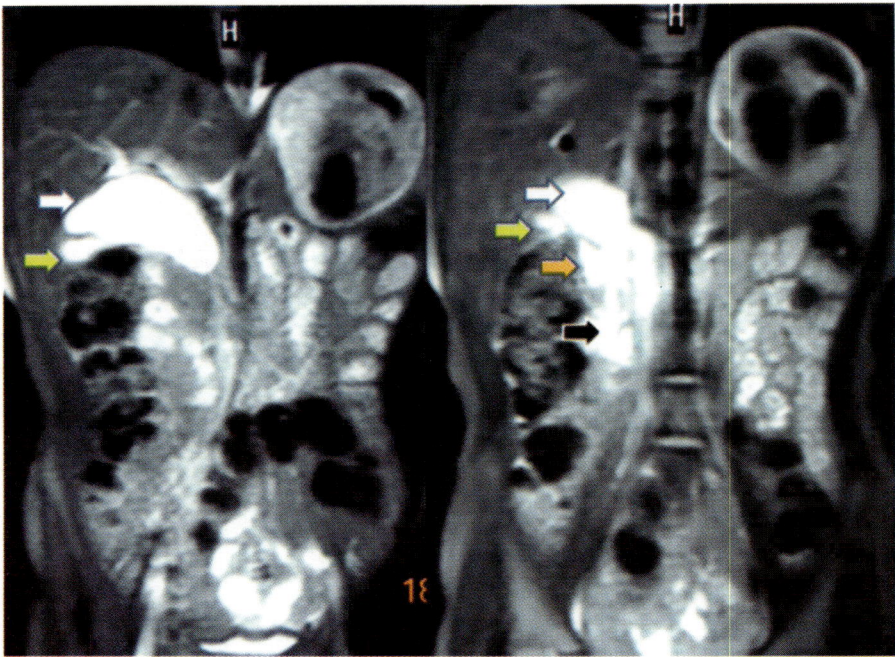

Fig. 4.15. MRCP images (coronal sections) showing type IA cyst (white arrows), gallbladder is shown by yellow, duodenum is shown by orange and bowel loops by black arrow.

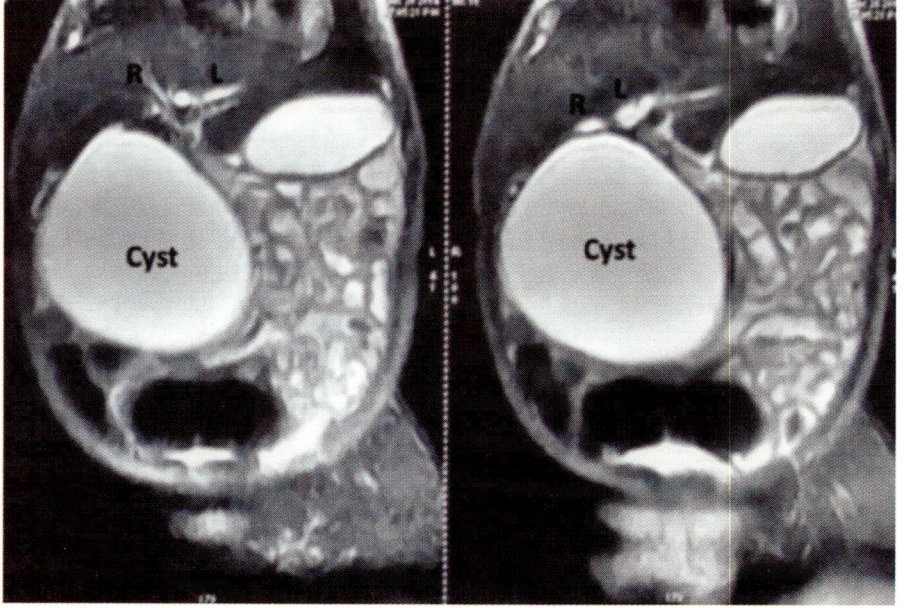

Fig. 4.16. MRCP images (coronal sections) showing a large type IA cyst with right and left hepatic ducts in a 1.5 month old female child.

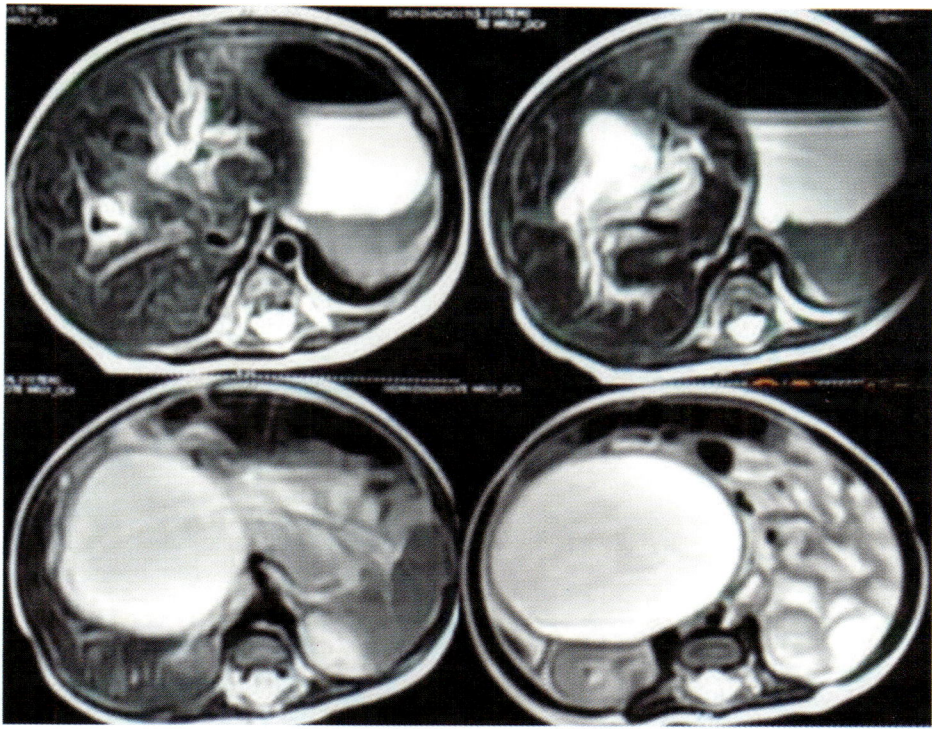

Fig. 4.17. MRCP images showing type IA cyst with dilated right and left hepatic ducts. The cyst was pushing both the hepatic ducts upwards and laterally in a 1.5 month old female child.

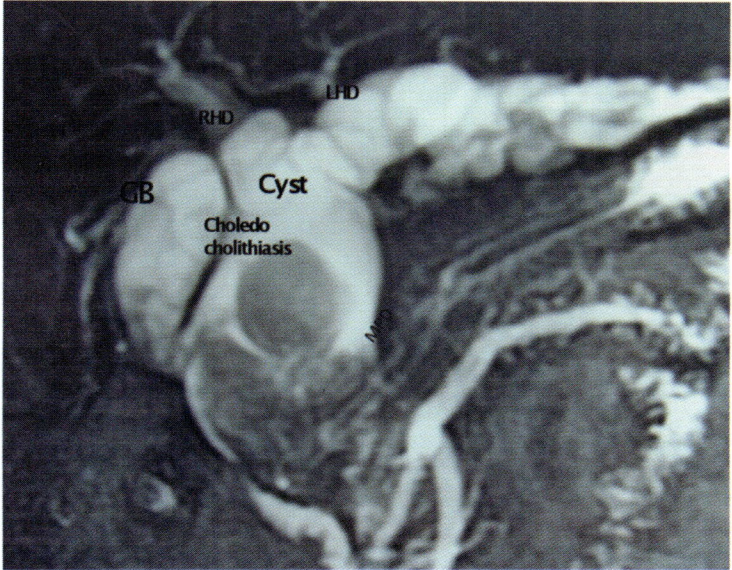

Fig. 4.18. MRCP images – type IVA cyst. Choledocholithiasis is seen.

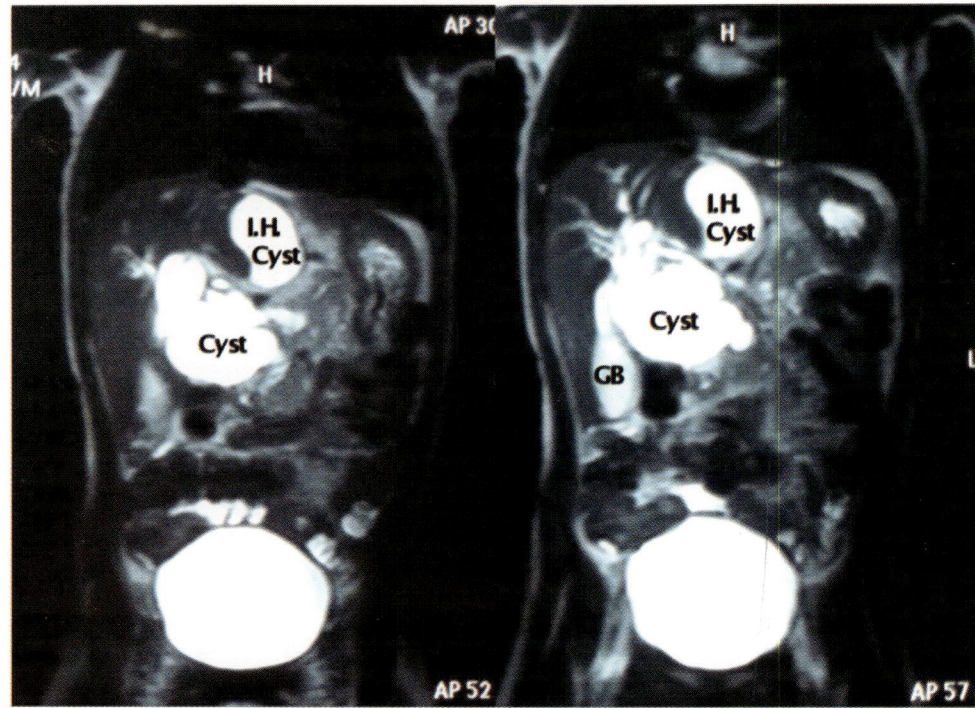

Fig. 4.19. MRCP images – type IVA cyst. I.H. Cyst – Intrahepatic cyst.

Choledochal Cyst Surgery

SURGICAL MANAGEMENT

PREOPERATIVE OPTIMIZATION

It is important. Preoperative correction of any bleeding tendency with either **parenteral vitamin K** administration or even fresh frozen plasma is a must. Intravenous (IV) antibiotics are given to treat any attack of cholangitis[24, 28].

TIMING OF SURGERY

Progressive intrahepatic ductal dilation, cyst enlargement, and deterioration of liver function are indications of obstruction and/or cholangitis, prompting early surgical intervention. **Also, a neonate with conjugated hyperbilirubinaemia and cystic dilatation of the biliary tree may possibly have a variant of extrahepatic biliary atresia which must be taken care by early surgery**[23]. It is believed that in asymptomatic patients, surgery should be performed within the first 3 months of age and we share this opinion, as it is observed that liver fibrosis progresses much faster in the neonates. Therefore, surgery should be performed early after diagnosis, even in asymptomatic prenatally diagnosed neonates, to prevent complications, particularly liver fibrosis.

In a neonate with a choledochal cyst, it takes 2 weeks or more for sludge to appear on ultrasound and result in obstructive jaundice, hence early correction at **2 weeks is advocated by researchers in antenatally diagnosed cases** to prevent the complications of liver fibrosis, proximal hepatic duct stenosis, hepatic dysfunction, cyst enlargement and perforation. Others believe that elective excision at 6 weeks is ideal. In any case the surgery should not be performed in haste and thorough assessment and planning is recommended.

Preoperative cyst drainage is warranted in severe cholangitis. It can be performed by percutaneous transhepatic biliary drainage, percutaneous cyst drainage, endoscopic internal drainage and T-tube drainage of the cyst.

PEROPERATIVE CHOLANGIOGRAPHY

Exploratory laparotomy with surgical (peroperative or intraoperative) cholangiography is recommended, being most informative. This is done by injecting contrast material through the gallbladder or cystic duct or directly into the choledochal cyst.

1. It helps in differentiating biliary atresia on the basis of the configuration of the intrahepatic bile ducts.
2. It provides accurate anatomical information regarding type of choledochal cyst.
3. Information regarding common channel and APBDJ.
4. Cystic dilatation may involve the retropancreatic portion in majority of cases. Pancreatic ductal opening may lie within the dilatation, and thus peroperative cholangiography may be extremely valuable in such cases.
5. Also reflux of contrast into intrahepatic ductal system determines presence of anomalous ducts/cysts or associated proximal intrahepatic ductal obstruction and calculi.

If cyst is very large, intraoperative cholangiography is not useful. In such cases, separate evaluation of intrahepatic biliary tree and distal CBD is performed at the end of cyst excision. It is not necessary if preoperative imaging undoubtedly visualizes the entire biliary tree and pancreatic duct.

OPERATIVE PROCEDURE

Historically, a cystenterostomy internal drainage procedure, cystoduodenostomy, cystojejunostomy, cystogastrostomy modified cystojejunostomy with T-tube external drainage, T-tube choledochocystomy with internal or external drainage, jejunal segment interposition with cystoduodenostomy were performed[7]. Choledochorrhaphy, that is, excision of the cyst wall and reconstruction of the bile duct, was abandoned due to high recurrence risk and non-alleviation of aetiological factors, so were bypass procedures involving anastomosis of gall-bladder to stomach, jejunum, or duodenum. Aspiration, marsupialization and external biliary drainage were also performed. Simple external biliary drainage procedures were unsuccessful due to long-standing external biliary fistula.

Cystenteric anastomosis is associated with an unacceptably high rate of late complications (60–70%), as it continues to stagnate bile despite an adequate biliary enteric stoma. Anastomotic stricture is secondary to the fact that the anastomosis should be performed as mucosa to mucosa, whereas the cyst does not have normal mucosa[7, 40]. Mucous lining shows inflammation, fibrosis and anastomotic site undergoes scarring leading to anastomotic stricture. The other late complications are secondary biliary calculus, recurrent cholangitis, hepatic abscess, biliary cirrhosis and risk of cholangiocarcinoma. Cyst internal drainage has been abandoned and total excision of the cyst and Roux-en-Y hepaticojejunostomy is recommended as the procedure of choice. **Also, the patients who had undergone previous cystenterostomy should be reoperated for complete resection of cyst and biliary diversion as early as possible.** In patients with postoperative biliary dysfunction after cyst internal drainage, there is strong indication for revision with cyst excision.

PRINCIPLES OF SURGERY

The most important rationale for aggressive management of choledochal cyst is the inherent possibility of malignancy. At present, the basic principle of management of choledochal cyst is excision of the entire dilated extrahepatic bile duct including the gallbladder, without damaging the adjacent vital structures such as portal vein, hepatic artery, pancreas and duodenum by meticulous dissection followed by biliary-enteric anastomosis. This procedure disconnects the pancreatic and biliary ducts. The most important rationale for aggressive management of choledochal cyst is the inherent risk of malignancy. The different types of anatomical variants of the hepatic arteries and the bile duct also increase the difficulty of surgery and increase the morbidity. These include anomalous hepatic arteries, accessory hepatic ducts, and primary ductal strictures. Therefore, meticulous dissection during surgery is paramount to prevent complications.

Cholecystectomy is always performed for all types of cyst:

1. Reflux and cholangitis are fewer when there is continuous bile flow.
2. Cholecystitis was observed on clinical and histological examination in patients in whom secondary operations were performed.
3. Reflux is well tolerated without cholangitis in those cases with cholecystectomy, complete excision of choledochal cyst and Roux-en-Y hepaticojejunostomy (bilio-enteric anastomosis).

The surgical management of choice for type I, type IVB and extrahepatic component of type IVA is complete excision of the involved portion of the extrahepatic bile duct from the hepatic hilum to the pancreaticobiliary duct junction with construction of a biliary-enteric anastomosis by a Roux-en-Y hepaticojejunostomy to restore continuity with the gastro-intestinal tract[40].

PROCEDURE OF CHOLEDOCHAL CYST EXCISION

Roof-top or a cheveron incision is made, with left limb smaller than the right limb (as shown in Fig. 5.1). Liver, spleen and pancreas are noted. Peritoneum over the cyst is incised transversely, cranial to the duodenum (Fig. 5.2). Gallbladder, which usually arises from the mid-portion of the choledochal cyst, should be dissected away from the hepatic bed. Cystic

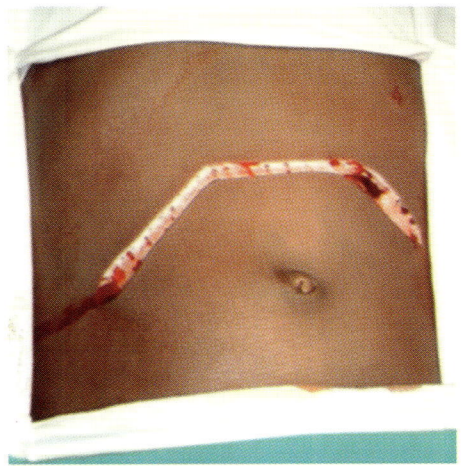

Fig. 5.1. Photograph showing bilateral subcostal incision (right > left for choledochal cyst).

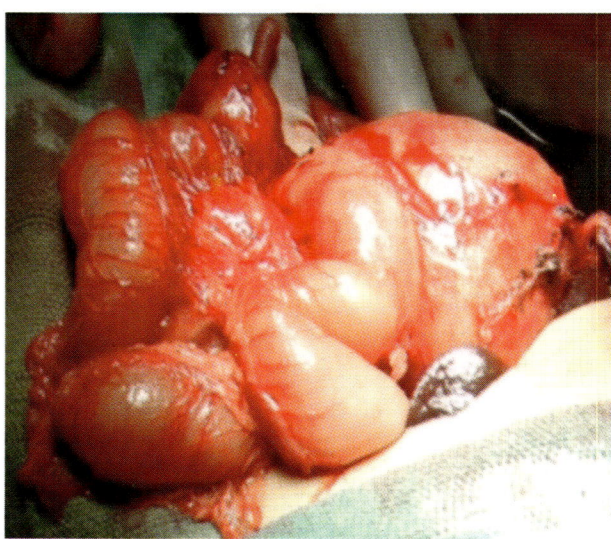

Fig. 5.2. On right: Intraoperative photograph taken from anesthetic end. The choledochal cyst is seen with close relation to duodenum.

artery is then carefully ligated. We perform this step early in the process because we believe that gentle and sustained traction on the gallbladder helps in dissection of the cyst from adherent structures (as a result of repeated inflammation) as shown in Figs. 5.3 & 5.4. Complete cyst excision is easier in young infants as wall of the cyst is thin and adhesions with surrounding viscera are minimal. In large and tense cyst, aspiration of cyst prior to dissection is rewarding. It should be sent for culture and biochemical (amylase and lipase) estimation.

Kocherisation is performed to expose the cyst (as low as possible) and then mobilization of cyst is performed carefully from the portal vein. Surgical cholangiography is performed at this stage, and particularly in those cases with unclear anatomy preoperatively. In large cysts outline of the distal duct and intrahepatic ducts may be obscured by direct injection into the cyst, so cholangiography is performed by contrast injection with butterfly needle into lower end of CBD and into CHD.

Plane of dissection should be close to the cyst wall. In case of chronic infection and recurrent inflammation there are periductal or pericystic adhesions, as a result dissection is easier said than done. Correct plane of dissection is easier at the hilar region in such cases. Combination of sharp and blunt dissection with use of bipolar cautery is recommended to achieve precise hemostasis. After the cyst has been exposed, gentle but sustained traction on the distal end of the cyst assists further dissection up to the pancreaticobiliary junction.

The goal is then to excise the intrapancreatic portion of the cyst without injuring the pancreatic duct or the long common channel. At this point, small vessels arising from the pancreas need careful cautery and ligation. The distal most portion of the choledochal cyst is encircled and transected at the level of caliber change or just proximal to the site where it enters the pancreatic duct (as shown in Figs. 5.5, 5.6, 5.7, 5.8, 5.9 & 5.10). In other words, division of cyst is done proximal to the pancreatic duct if it is seen or identified or as low as

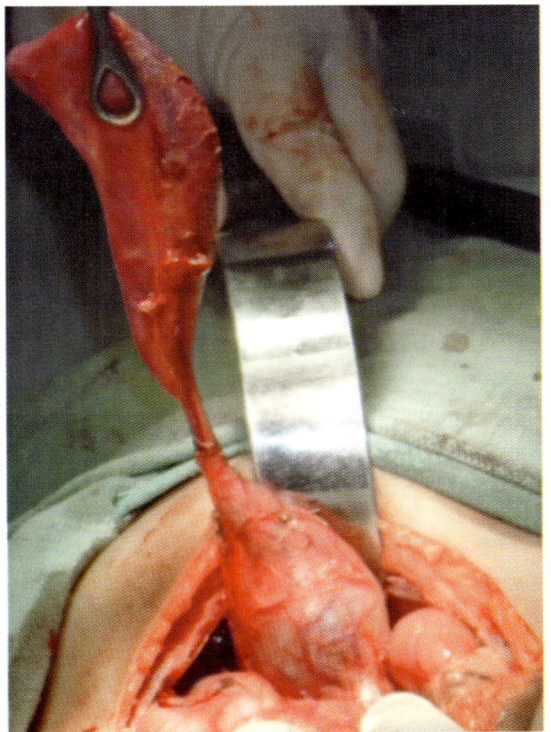

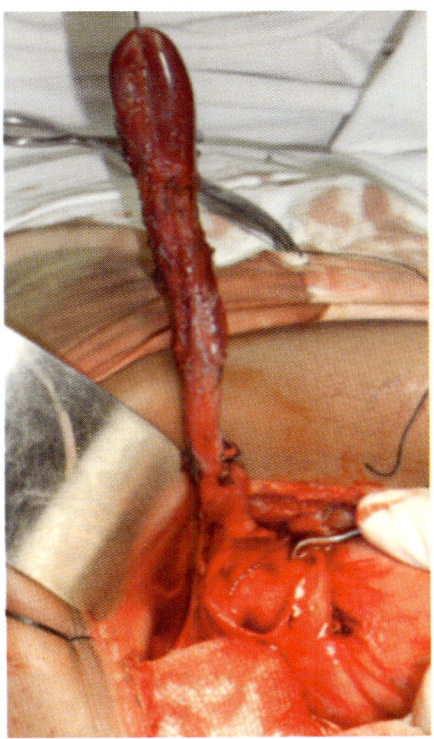

Fig. 5.3. Intraoperative photograph showing chole-dochal cyst, with gallbladder removed from hepatic bed and used for gentle traction for easing the dissection of the cyst taken from anesthetic end.

Fig. 5.4. Intraoperative photograph showing choledochal cyst which has been opened from its anterior wall.

possible for the reason that remnant tissue will lead to reformation of cyst or a diverticulum. This will further lead to recurrent pancreatitis, calculi formation or malignancy in residual cyst or diverticulum. Distal CBD is closed by suturing. If the choledochal cyst extends distally into the pancreas, the mucosa of the intrapancreatic portion of the cyst should be stripped away prior to closure at the point of distal transection. Theoretically, this removes the risk of malignant transformation in that segment of the duct. Any protein plug, stone debris in the common channel is flushed or removed to prevent postoperative complications. The distal bile duct stump should be double-suture ligated with polydioxanone or silk suture.

Gentle and sustained traction on the gallbladder and the cyst helps in exposing the portal vein from behind. Few authors recommend opening of the cyst in its anterior wall in all the cases. We perform cystotomy in only those cases with marked adhesions (Fig. 5.11).

Occasionally **right hepatic artery** crosses in front of the cyst and may be adherent to its wall. It should be meticulously preserved. Cyst is transected at the level of distinct caliber change (as shown in Fig. 5.12) or at the bifurcation of the CHD or more proximally if it extends into the individual hepatic ducts (as shown in Figs. 5.13, 5.14 A & B). This place meant for biliary-enteric anastomosis should be healthy and vascularised. The reason for removal of proximal cyst mucosa is due to its tendency for malignant degeneration.

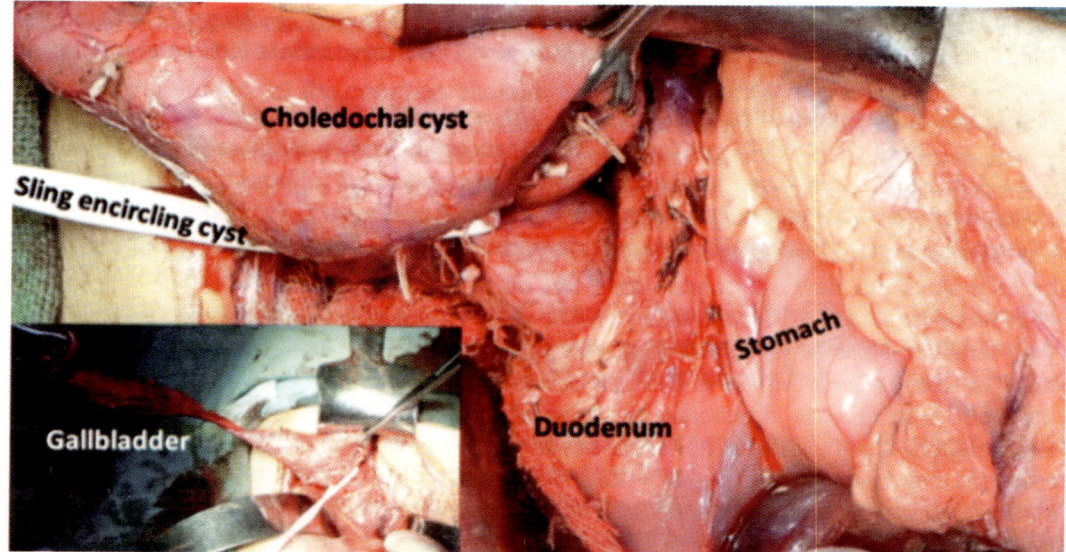

Fig. 5.5. Intraoperative photograph showing the lower end of the cyst which has been dissected circumferentially.

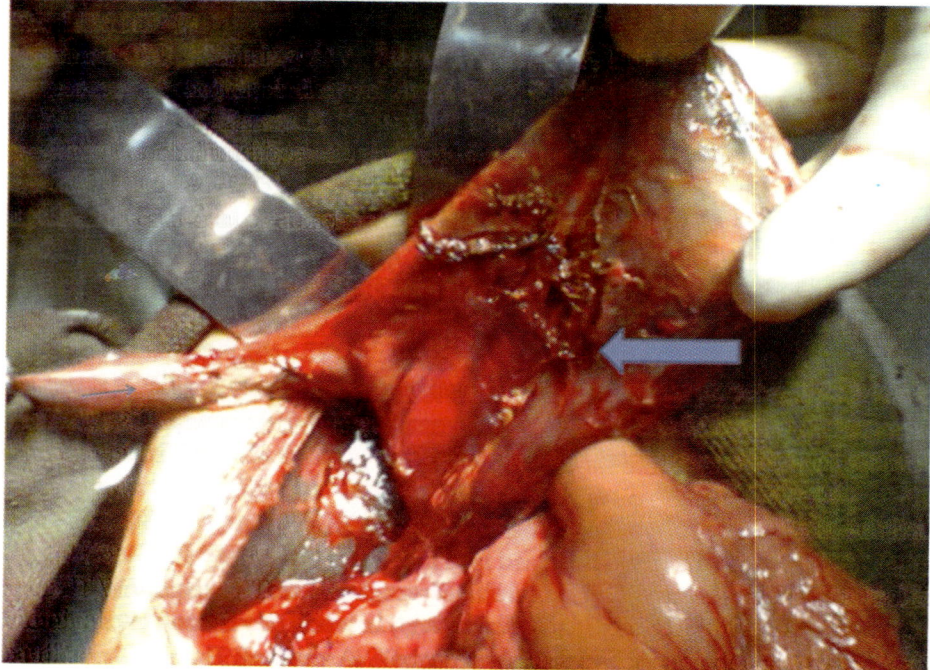

Fig. 5.6. Peroperative photograph of type IA choledochal cyst (blue arrow), with the gallbladder (blue line). The cyst has been dissected from the surrounding structures along with the gallbladder removed from the gallbladder bed (cholecystectomy).

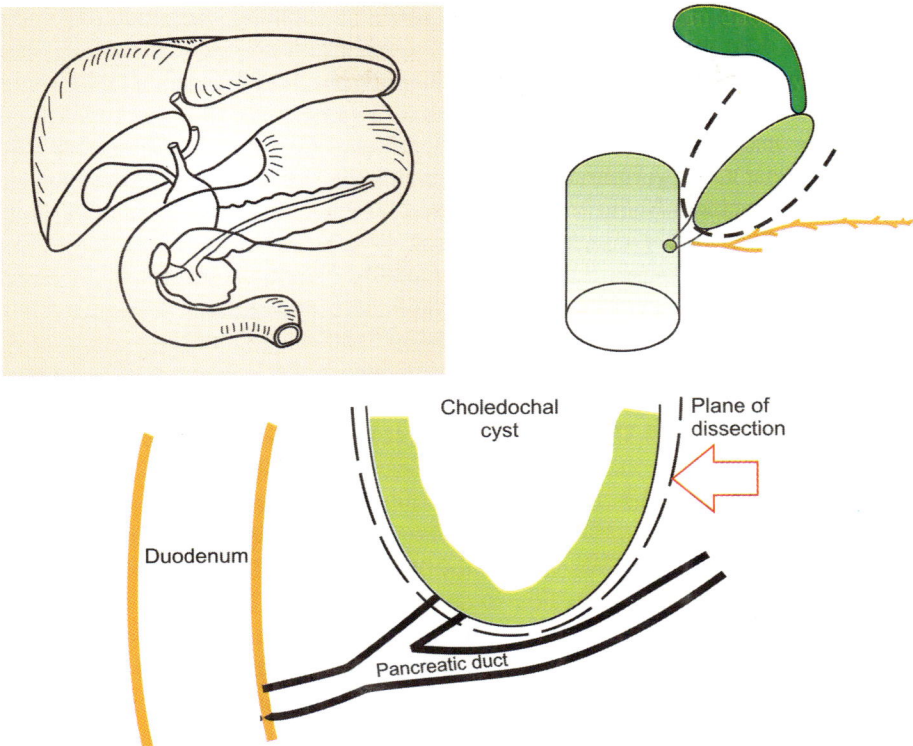

Figs. 5.7, 5.8 & 5.9. Diagrammatic representation to show type IA choledochal cyst, biliary anatomy and long common channel. Plane of dissection at lower end of choledochal cyst is presented. The cyst is cut just proximal to pancreatic duct opening.

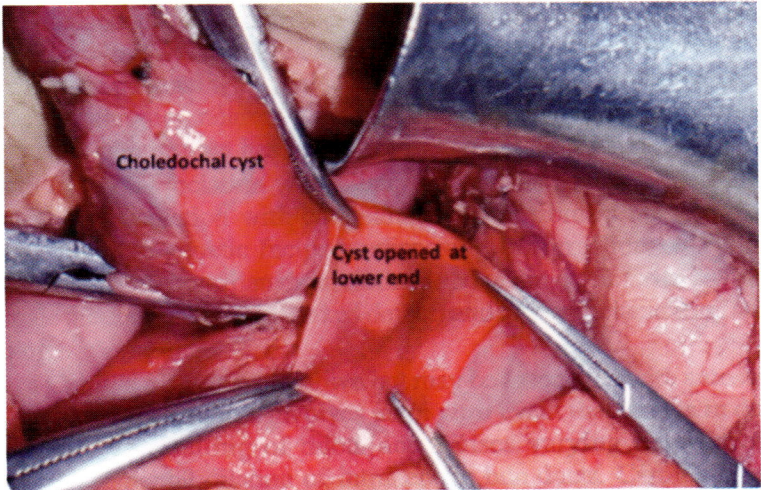

Fig. 5.10. Peroperative photograph showing cut lower end of choledochal cyst to demonstrate its opening into the duodenum.

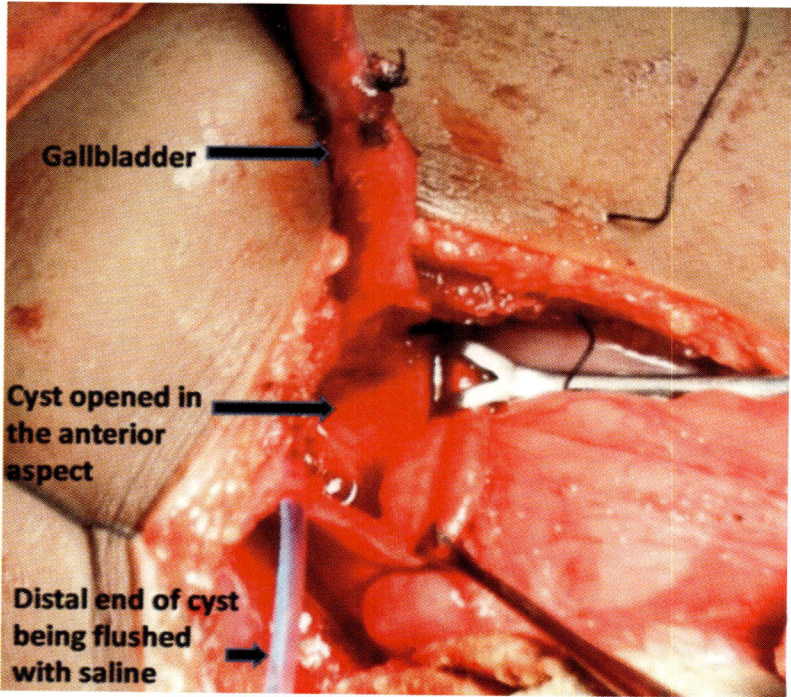

Fig. 5.11. Peroperative photograph of type IA choledochal cyst which was opened at its anterior wall. Its lower and upper ends being flushed with normal saline.

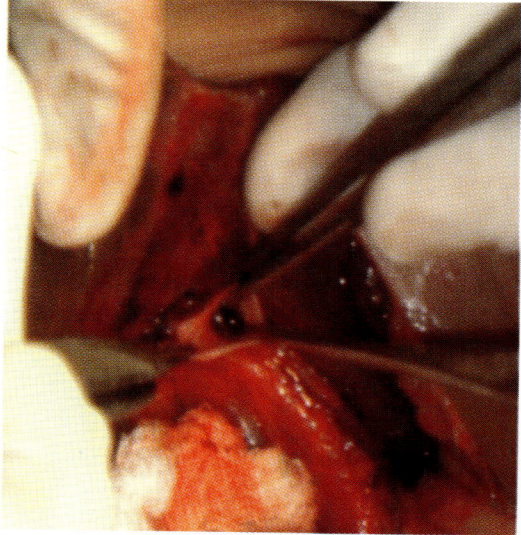

Fig. 5.12. Peroperative photograph showing CHD prepared for Roux-en-Y HJ, after cyst excision.

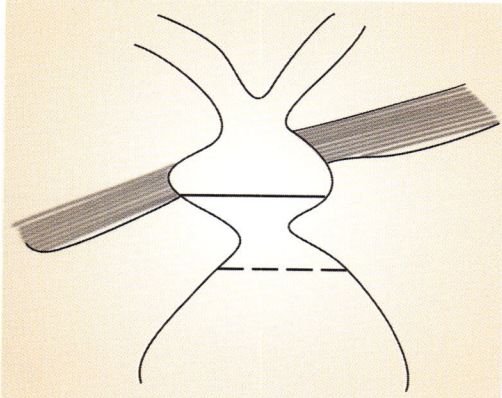

Fig. 5.13. Diagrammatic representation to show level of excision (upper line) above the level of stricture. Dotted line represents the wrong level.

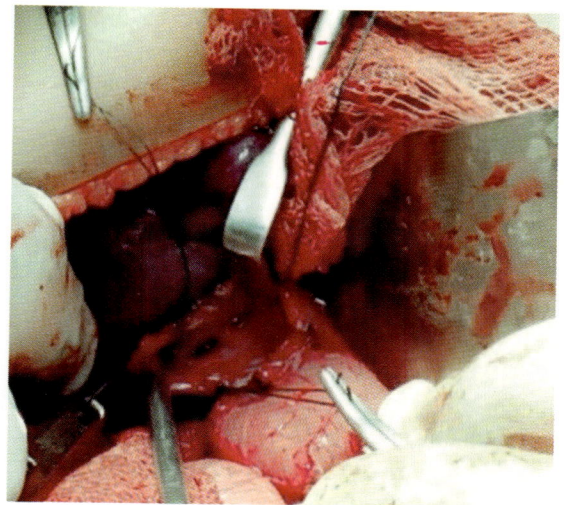

Fig. 5.14A. Peroperative photograph showing the common hepatic duct prepared for Roux-en-Y hepaticojejunostomy, both right and left hepatic ducts are seen.

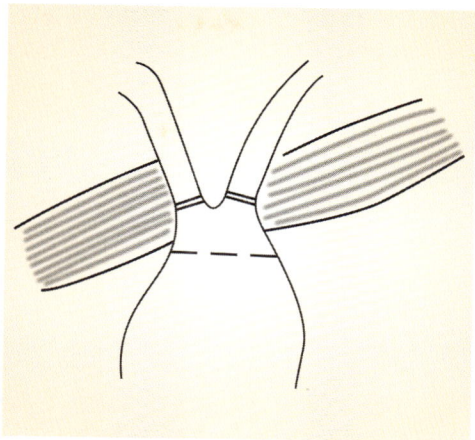

Fig. 5.14B. Diagrammatic representation to show level of excision (upper lines) as cyst is extending above the level of confluence of right and left hepatic ducts. Dotted line represents the wrong level.

In type IVA cyst, transection of CHD is done at the confluence of the cyst.

After excision of the cyst, the intrahepatic ducts should be probed and lavaged with saline to disencumber the ductal system of sludge and possible stones. If not taken care at this time, stones can lead to recurrent pancreatitis, and pain abdomen. Additionally, on occasion, obstruction may be found in the proximal biliary system, which can be dilated. Therefore, intraoperative cholangiography before cyst excision is a valuable investigation.

Dilatation of peripheral IHBD in patients with type IA choledochal cyst may be associated with recurrent cholangitis, anastomotic strictures, and stone formation. These complications are rare in younger patients. Excessive intervention is not recommended.

Dissection of posterior layer of the cyst and dissection of the distal part of the cyst from the head of the pancreas are the most difficult parts of the entire procedure.

In **type II complete excision of the dilated diverticulum**, the resultant defect in the common bile duct is closed over a T-tube. If the defect/base of the cyst is wide, then treat as per type I.

Therapeutic choice depends on the size of the cyst in type III. Endoscopic treatment is the method of choice for uncomplicated cyst. Choledochoceles measuring 3 cm or less can be treated effectively with endoscopic sphincterotomy, whereas lesions larger than 3 cm (which typically produce some degree of duodenal obstruction) are excised surgically or transduodenal sphincteroplasty is performed.

SURGICAL PROCEDURE FOR TYPE III CYST

After Kocherisation is performed, a longitudinal duodenotomy permits complete exposure of an intraduodenal choledochocele. Once the choledochocele is exposed, a small aperture is made to drain the bile on the surface of the lesion. An intraoperative cholangiogram is performed. Choledochocele should be unroofed, and then the marsupialisation (mucosa is reapproximated) is performed with multiple interrupted absorbable sutures. Openings of CBD and MPD are calibrated (as they may be narrow) to justify sphincteroplasty. If the pancreatic duct enters the choledochocele, its reimplantation into the duodenum may be required following excision of the cyst[40]. Rarely pancreaticoduodenectomy may be required. Although carcinoma may rarely coexist with choledochocele, but measures, such as endoscopic ultrasonography and biopsy, may be required to exclude malignancy.

Intrahepatic dilatation of type IVA cyst in children does not adversely affect the post-operative outcome after conventional surgical repair. These intrahepatic dilatations are always left-sided, but right-sided cysts may coexist. It has been suggested that fusiform type of dilatation of the intrahepatic biliary radicles (IHBR) is related to sustained increase of intra-biliary pressure rather than any intrinsic intrahepatic cystic malformation and that effective surgery invariably reduces measured intrahepatic dilatation towards normal values[41]. Cystic IHBR dilatation may be a primary abnormality. Management options include conservative approach (especially in fusiform type), segmentectomy, partial hepatectomy, balloon dilatation of the stenoses, and intrahepatic cystoenterostomy. In type IVA intrahepatic ductal disease resection of the affected hepatic segment or lobe is indicated in hepatolithiasis, intrahepatic ductal strictures, and hepatic abscesses. In localized intrahepatic ductal disease relevant partial hepatectomy may be performed due to risk of malignancy[41].

Inclusion of the proximal end of the CHD in the excision is essential for favourable long-term results following surgical procedure in type IV cyst. There is often a membranous or septal stenosis of the hepatic ducts at their confluence in type IV cyst, which can contribute to biliary stasis and formation of intrahepatic calculi.

In type V, preferred treatment remains controversial. It is difficult to treat because of predisposition to severe recurrent cholangitis, and subsequent biliary cirrhosis. Both conservative and surgical modalities are undertaken and frequent follow-up is required in these patients. Hepatic lobectomy for disease limited to one hepatic lobe and liver trans-plantation for bilobar disease, diffuse hepatic fibrosis, hepatolithiasis with repeated cholangitis, secondary biliary cirrhosis, liver failure and portal hypertension are treatment options[40].

In the absence of cirrhosis or malignancy, Roux-en-Y hepaticojejunostomy with bilateral transhepatic silastic stents may be indicated to improve biliary drainage (stents left for 6–12 months). In cases with either a part or whole of the intrahepatic component is left, an access loop of the jejunum is created with the Roux-en-Y limb. It would endow a simple method for removal of intrahepatic biliary sludge, calculi or debris endoscopically. The access loop can be either placed subcutaneously or created as duodenojejunal anastomosis. The rare indication is when the excision of functioning hepatic parenchyma would be either unnecessary or contraindicated.

Cholecystectomy with cystic duct ligation near the common bile duct is curative in type VI. Liver biopsy is taken to evaluate the degree of cirrhosis. Excised cyst should be examined grossly for malignancy and should be sent for frozen section.

In patients with biliary peritonitis following perforation of choledochal cyst, severe cholangitis, poor hemodynamic condition, initially external biliary drainage, with subsequent delayed primary cyst excision 1 to 2 month later is recommended. Preliminary external biliary drainage of the cyst with T-tube or percutaneous hepaticostomy can help detect the presence of distal biliary calculus or protein plugs or any obstruction prior to the definitive procedure.

INTRAOPERATIVE ENDOSCOPY

Intraoperative endoscopy of the common channel, intrahepatic biliary ducts, and pancreatic duct, using a fine fiberoptic scope or paediatric choledochoscope or cystoscope can help in detection as well as management of protein plugs, debris and stones. It can also detect intrahepatic dilatations, and strictures at the junction of the intrahepatic ducts and common hepatic duct, and APBDJ. It helps in evaluation of level of transection of the CHD. Japanese group recommends a more fine and flexible neonatal cystoscope with a flush channel for diagnostic as well as therapeutic purpose (Fig. 5.15).

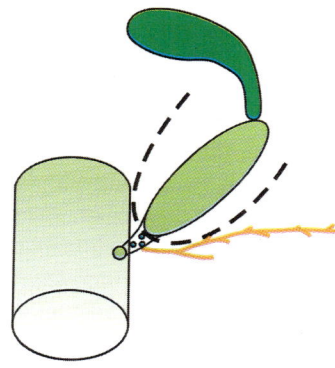

Fig. 5.15. Diagrammatic representation to show sludge, protein plugs, debris and nidus for calculi in the distal end. Dotted line represents the plane of dissection. Hence lies the importance of intraoperative endoscopy which can guide the operating surgeon to decide the level of transaction at lower end, identify pancreatic duct orifice, and prevents its injury. Also it can prevent reformation of the cyst due to residual cyst, if transaction is done at higher level.

ROUX-EN-Y PROCEDURE

Before embarking upon biliary reconstruction or biliary enteric continuity we would like to mention few words about Roux-en-Y and pay our obeisance to César Roux.

Roux-en-Y is pronounced as rôô'ìn-wî'. Roux' procedure (Roux-en-Y procedure) is a common method of using small intestines as a means to re-route gastrointestinal secretions or food and maintain (retain) the continuity of the gastrointestinal tract. Small bowel i.e. jejunum is divided roughly 15–30 cm distal to the duodenojejunal junction and anastomosis of the distal divided end is performed to the stomach, oesophagus, biliary tract (CHD) or pancreatic duct. Anastomosis of the proximal end is done to the side of the jejunum at a suitable distance, approximately 40 cm below the anastomosis.

Roux' procedure is named after César Roux (1857–1934), a Swiss surgeon, who originally described this technique in 1893. César Roux worked under Christopher Theodor Aeby and Theodor Langhans. He was greatly inspired by Emil Theodor Kocher, Theodor Billroth and Richard von Volkmann. He initially performed this procedure in a patient of G.O.O. (Gastric

Outlet Obstruction) following chronic peptic ulcer. Stick figure representation of the bowel arrangement forms a Y-shaped pattern. Thus to honour César Roux and with the vague similarity with letter "Y", it is named as Roux-en-Y procedure.

Table 5.1. Indications of Roux-en-Y procedure
1. Gastric substitution (gastric cancer, GOO)
2. Oesophageal substitution (oesophageal atresia, oesophageal malignancy)
3. Biliary duct obstruction (choledochal cyst, CBD and CHD strictures, benign or malignant)
4. CBD or CHD tumour (cholangiocarcinoma)
5. Biliary atresia
6. Periampullary carcinoma
7. Chronic pancreatitis
8. Pancreatic pseudocyst
9. Pancreas reconstruction after blunt abdominal trauma
10. Pancreas transplant
11. Bariatric surgery, a treatment for morbid obesity

BILIARY RECONSTRUCTION

The choice of intestinal conduit should be technically simple and prevent reflux. The 40 cm Roux-en-Y jejunal limb is most acceptable. Roux-en-Y hepaticojejunostomy is the "gold standard" procedure for biliary reconstruction in choledochal cyst (Fig. 5.16). Biliary reconstruction should be performed as high as possible, near the hilum of the liver, by using the jejunum at a distance of about 15 to 30 cm, cutting the jejunum from ligament of Treitz

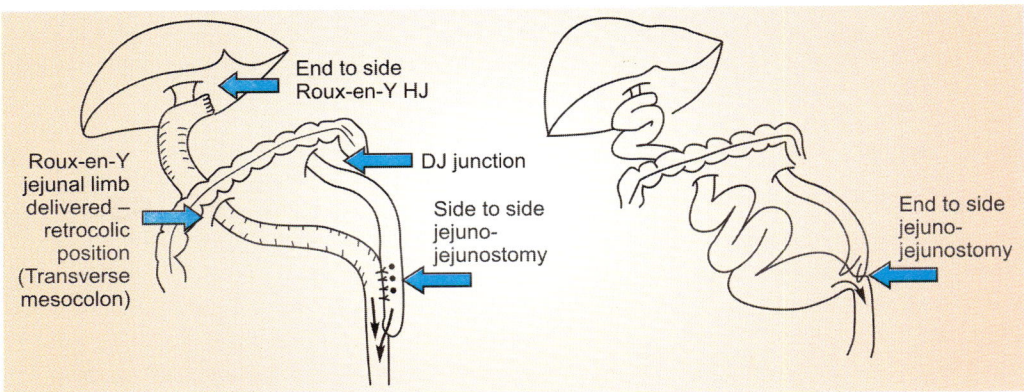

Fig. 5.16. Diagrammatic representation of end to side Roux-en-Y hepaticojejunostomy (HJ). The 40 cm Roux-en-Y jejunal limb is prepared, after transecting the jejunum 15–30 cm from the duodenojejunal junction (DJ) and delivered into the hilar region of the liver with retrocolic position. Top figure: Jejunal limb from ligament of Treitz & Roux limb is approximated side to side. Bottom figure: End to side jejunojejunal (T-shaped) anastomosis which is not preferred because of unusual dilatation of bile draining limb of jejunum as a result of reflux of jejunal contents into Roux limb which obstructs the flow of bile.

(duodenojejunal flexure). Jejunum is transected only after visualization and preservation of the vascular arcade of the jejunum (as shown in Fig. 5.17). Distal jejunum is closed (as shown in Fig. 5.18). The 40 cm Roux-en-Y jejunal limb is prepared (30 cm in infants) and delivered into the hilar region of the liver with retrocolic position (through transverse mesocolon and to the right of middle colic vessels) as shown in Fig. 5.18. 40 cm is sufficient length for effectively preventing reflux. 30 cm limb is required in infants because intestine is expected to lengthen with age of the child. Redundancy of the Roux-en-Y limb is likely to occur with larger lengths and it should be individualised. Redundancy of the Roux-en-Y limb will lead to biliary stasis, which may further lead to repeated bouts of cholangitis and its complications.

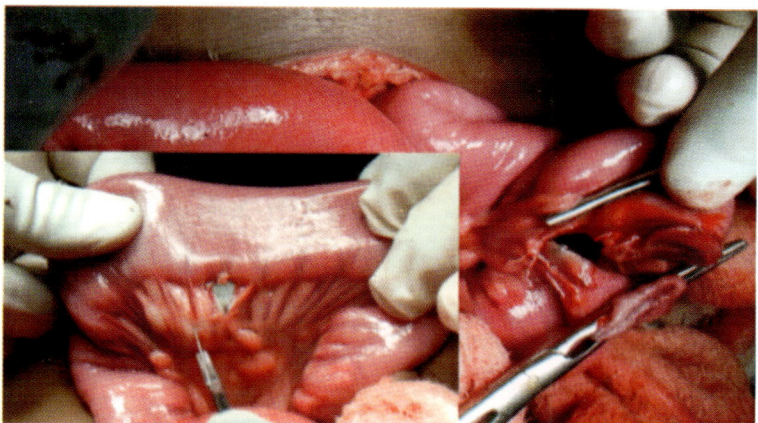

Fig. 5.17. Peroperative photograph showing jejunum being transected 15 cm from duodenojejunal flexure (15 to 30 cm), carefully preserving the vascular arcade.

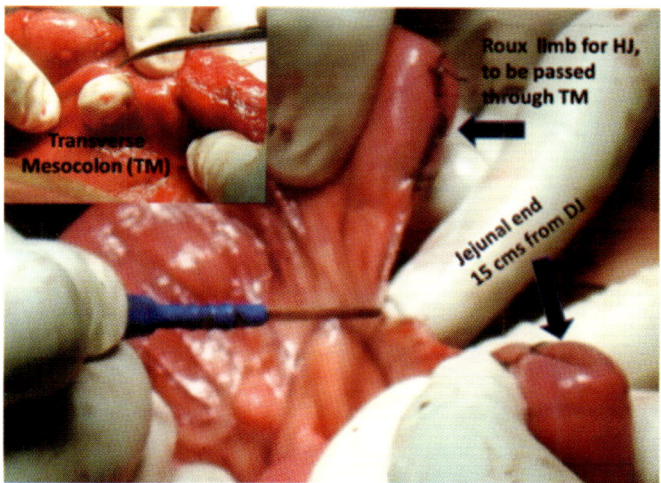

Fig. 5.18. Peroperative photograph showing jejunum being prepared for HJ (hepaticojejunostomy) after closing both the ends. Transverse mesocolon is opened to deliver the Roux limb retrocolically near the hepatic hilum.

The conduit is opened at antimesenteric border just proximal (not few cm) to closed jejunal end (as shown in Fig. 5.19) and then end to side anastomosis between common hepatic duct (CHD) and jejunum is done with interrupted, absorbable, monofilament sutures (Polydioxanone) (Figs. 5.20, 5.21, 5.22, 5.23, 5.24, 5.25 & 5.26). If CHD at hepatic hilum is narrow, the left and right hepatic ducts can be slit open for a few millimetres so as to achieve a wide anastomosis (as shown in Figs. 5.23 & 5.24). Anastomosis to narrow CHD should be avoided to prevent long-term risk of anastomotic stricture.

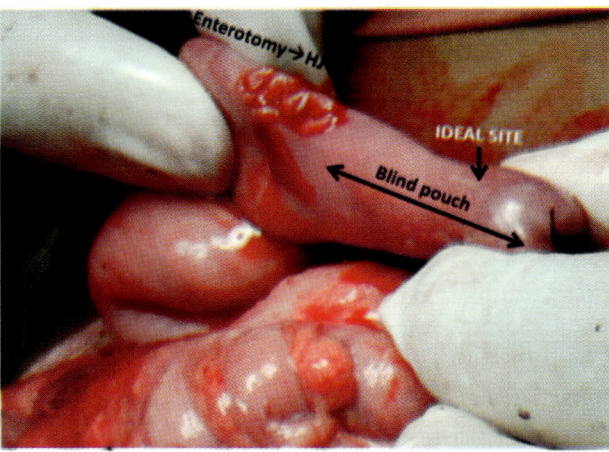

Fig. 5.19. Peroperative photograph showing jejunum being prepared for HJ (hepaticojejunostomy) after closing both the ends. Transverse mesocolon is opened to deliver the Roux limb retrocolically near the hepatic hilum.

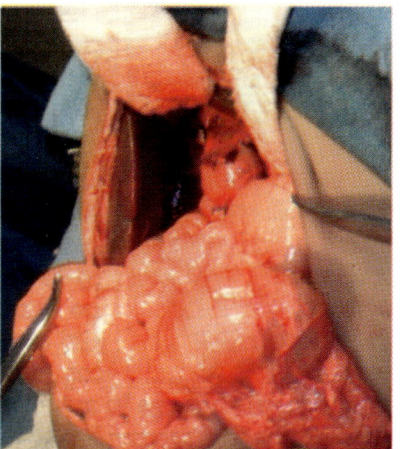
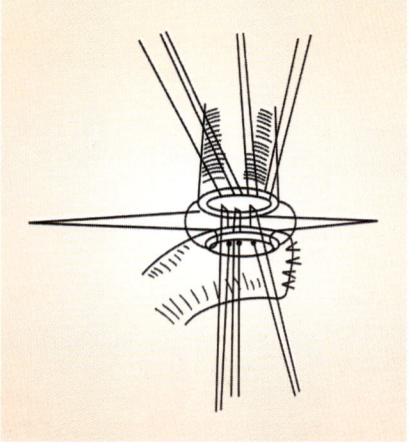

Fig. 5.20. Peroperative photograph showing end to side Roux-en-Y hepaticojejunostomy being performed. Inset image shows creation of end to side HJ. Anterior rows of sutures on the bile duct are inserted first and elevated along with needles. The posterior rows of sutures are then placed through the bowel as well, then jejunum is railroaded upwards in proximity to CHD and sutures are tied. Anterior row of sutures is finally tied.

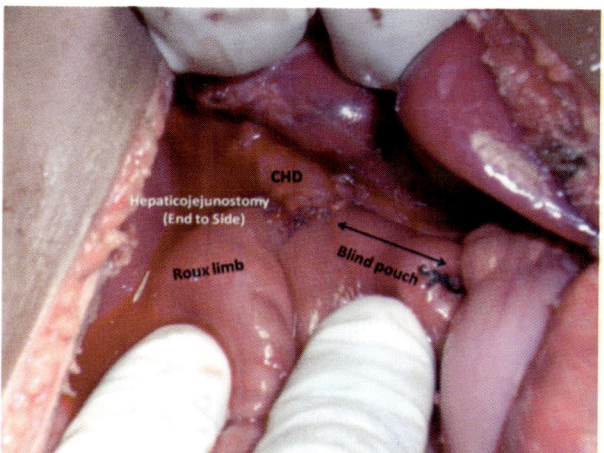 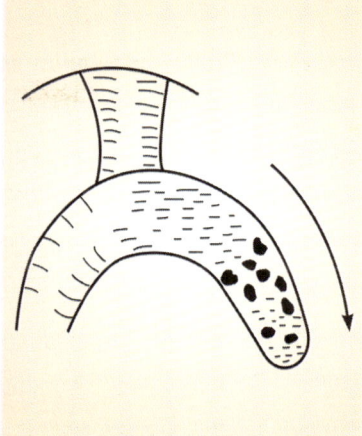

Fig. 5.21. Peroperative photograph showing Roux-en-Y hepaticojejunostomy. Anastomosis has been performed away from the closed jejunal end which will result in blind pouch. Inset image shows end to side Roux-en-Y hepaticojejunostomy away from the closed jejunal end resulting in formation of blind pouch and its complications of stone formation and biliary stasis.

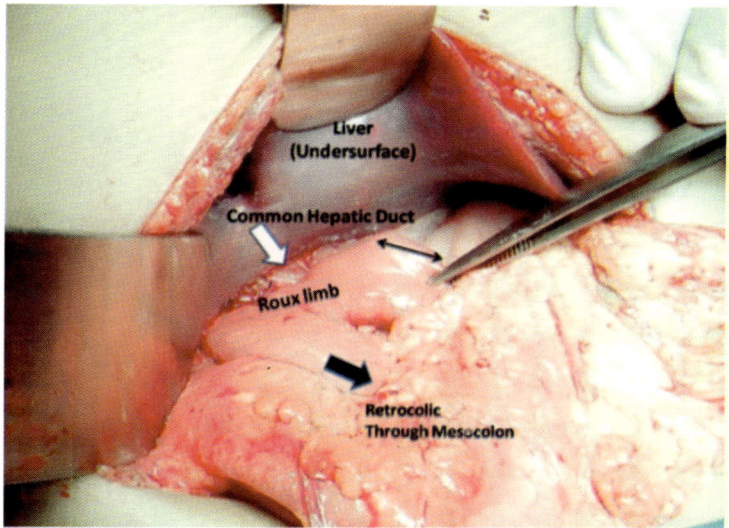

Fig. 5.22. Peroperative photograph showing completion of end to side Roux-en-Y hepaticojejunostomy. Arrow shows distance of anastomosis from blind end.

Sushruta describes surgery –

'... the 1st and highest division of the healing art ... superior in producing instantaneous effects ... least liable to fallacy, pure in itself, perpetual in its applicability, the worthy produce of heaven, and the sure source of fame on Earth.'

Nonetheless, Sushruta quickly admonishes against forgetting one's knowledge of medicine for 'He who only knows one branch of his art, is like a bird with one wing'.

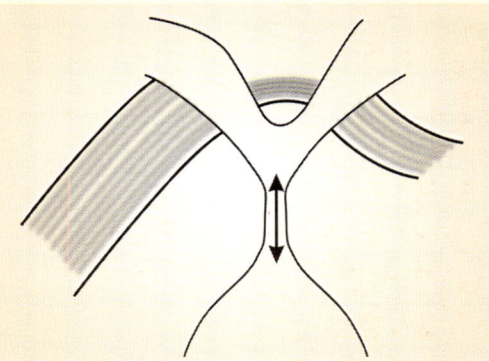

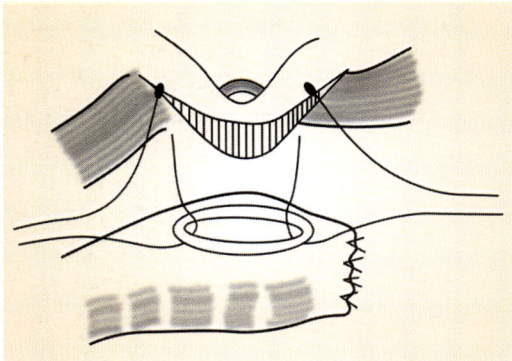

Fig. 5.23. Diagrammatic representation to show choledochal cyst with stenosis of the CHD. Arrow showing extent of stenosis.

Fig. 5.24. HJ at hepatic hilum after creating wide stoma made by making incisions along the lateral wall of the CHD, right and left ducts.

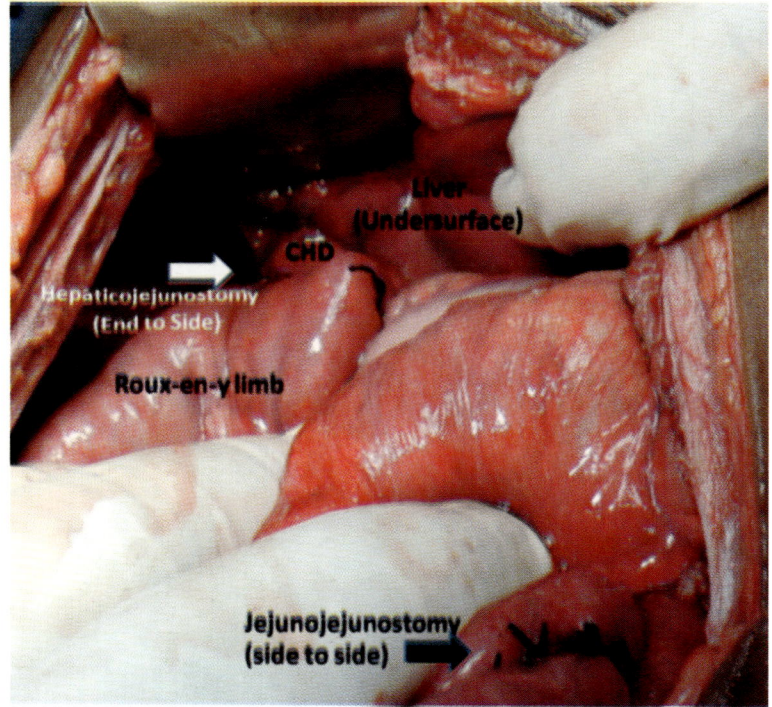

Fig. 5.25. Peroperative photograph showing end to side Roux-en-Y hepaticojejunostomy (white arrow) just near the blind end.

150 people die every year from being hit by falling coconuts. Not to worry, drug makers are developing a vaccine.

Jim Carrey

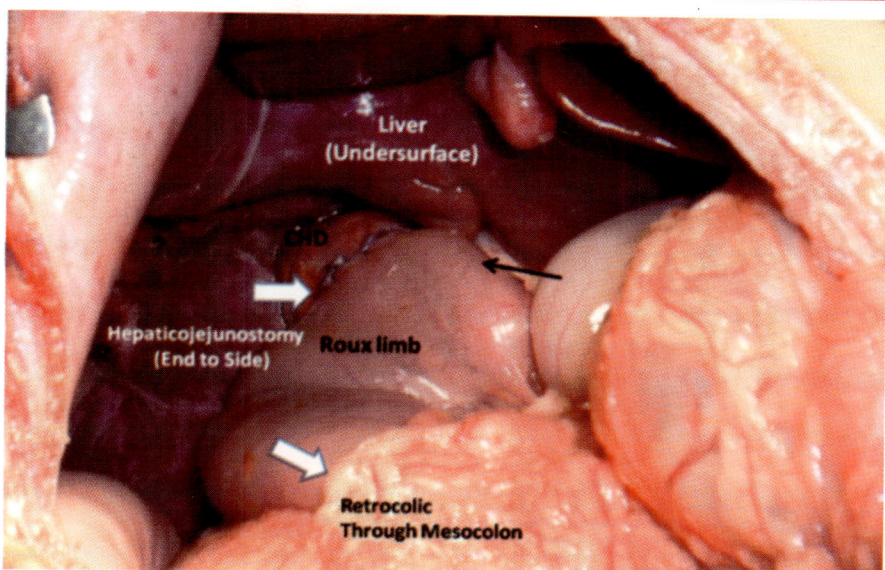

Fig. 5.26. Peroperative photograph showing end to side Roux-en-Y hepaticojejunostomy just near the blind end.

Hepaticojejunostomy at hepatic hilum (Fig. 5.24) is indicated in patients with dilated intrahepatic bile duct with stenosis in CHD. It is a challenging technique, particularly in infants, where there is absence of intrahepatic bile duct dilatation. Hilar ductal strictures require ductoplasty or extended anastomosis.

End to end anastomosis (Fig. 5.27) of jejunum to the upper end of remnant (hepatico-jejunostomy) is recommended if ratio of CHD diameter and proximal Roux limb of jejunum is < 1 : 2.5 (CHD : jejunum). End to end anastomosis is also recommended by Japanese group as with this technique, drainage is direct and smooth. They report overgrowth of the blind end (as shown in Fig. 5.21) in later life as child grows, bile stasis in blind pouch leading to bowel obstruction and stone formation in pouch. We routinely perform end to side hepaticojejunostomy close to the end of Roux limb to prevent blind pouch in our institution. We occasionally place a gelfoam near our anastomosis for preventing peri-anastomotic bleeding (ooze) as shown in Fig. 5.28.

Intestinal continuity is restored by a Roux-en-Y end to side jejunojejunostomy (as shown in Fig. 5.29) or a Roux-en-Y side to side jejunojejunostomy (as shown in Figs. 5.30 & 5.31). Length of the Roux-en-Y limb should be such that the Roux-en-Y jejunojejunostomy fits naturally into the splenic flexure and returns back into the peritoneal cavity after jejuno-jejunostomy. Jejunal limb from ligament of Treitz and Roux limb should be approximated side to side for about 8 cm proximally in case of end to side anastomosis to ensure smooth flow of bile. Without this the anastomosis will become T-shaped and there may be reflux of jejunal contents into the Roux limb, with the resultant complications of biliary stasis. Mesenteric defects in transverse mesocolon and small bowel mesentery are closed. Liver biopsy is performed for histopathological evaluation. An abdominal drain is kept in Morison's pouch after abdominal toileting.

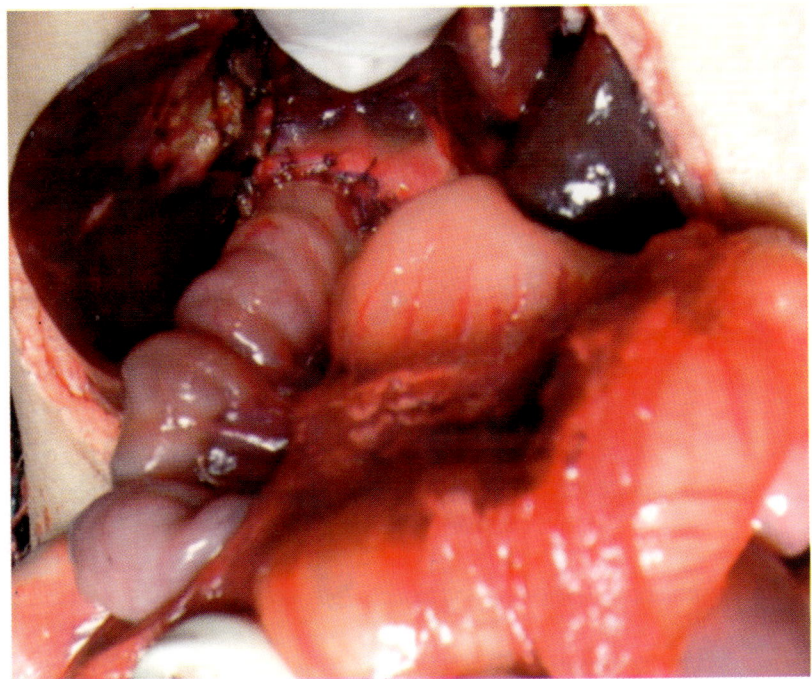

Fig. 5.27. Peroperative photograph showing end to end Roux-en-Y hepaticojejunostomy.

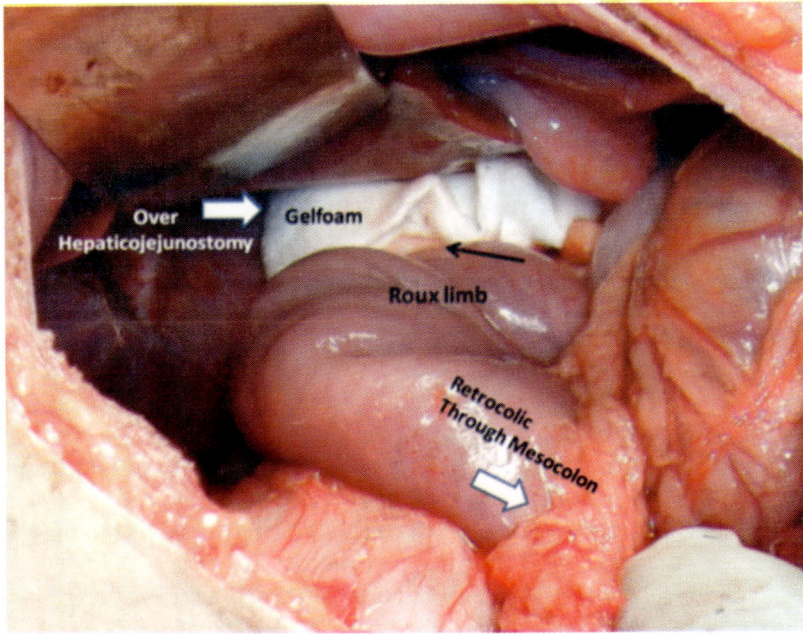

Fig. 5.28. Peroperative photograph showing gelfoam applied over Roux-en-Y hepaticojejunostomy.

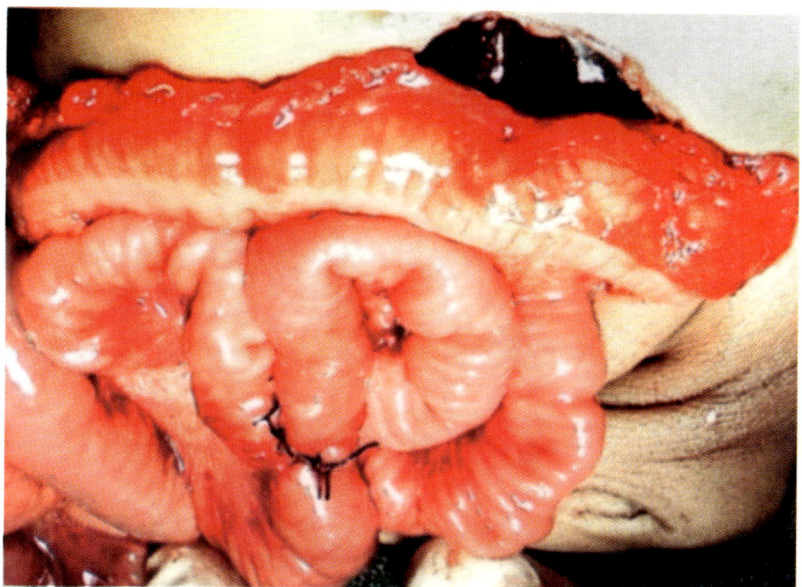

Fig. 5.29. Peroperative photograph showing end to side jejunojejunostomy. Both limbs are approximated side to side for few cm proximally to prevent obstruction of Roux limb.

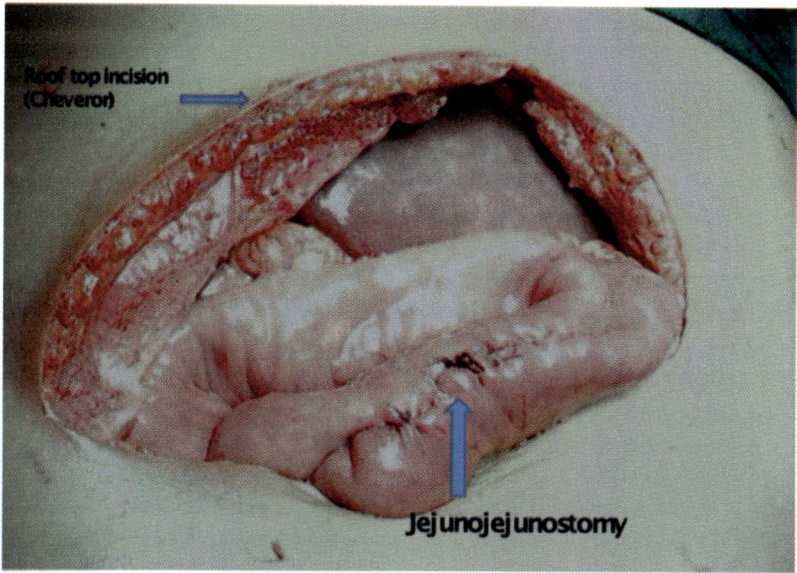

Fig. 5.30. Peroperative photograph showing completion of side to side jejunojejunostomy.

God heals and the Physician hath the thankes.
George Herbert

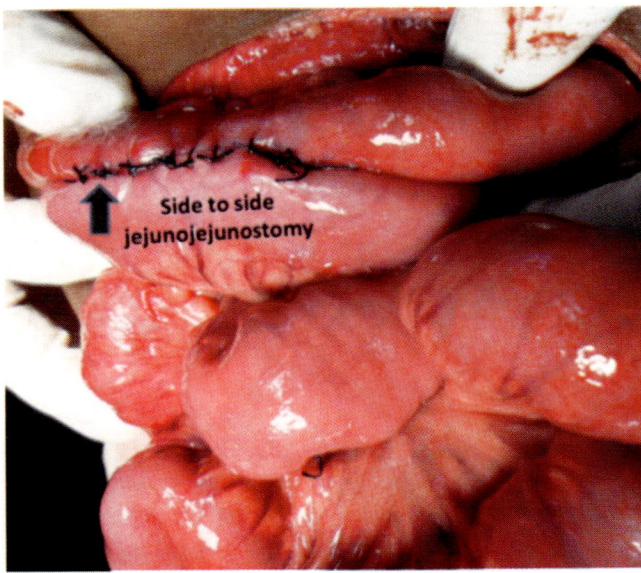

Fig. 5.31. Peroperative photograph showing completion of side to side jejunojejunostomy.

LILLY'S PROCEDURE

In patients with recurrent bouts of cholangitis, and pericystic inflammation, the cyst adheres densely to the portal vein and adjacent vascular structures (Figs. 5.32 & 5.33). This is true, especially in the older children, adults and those with cystic type of choledochal cyst. In these cases periductal or pericystic dissection with full-thickness excision of the cyst is unsafe owing to the dreaded complication of portal venous injury, in particular. Prior to dissection of the cyst in these cases, opening of anterior wall of the cyst is recommended. The posterior wall of the cyst is now directly seen from inside. Excision is then accomplished by removing only the less adherent portion. The posterior wall is dissected using a plane between the inner (mucosa) and outer layers of the cyst (serosal surface) or mucosa of the cyst wall is obliterated by curettage or cautery. Hence, the portion of the cyst wall and bile duct that is adherent to the portal vein and hepatic artery is left undisturbed. This is Lilly's procedure, also known as Lilly's mucosectomy technique[42–43]. It can be performed with laparoscopic technique also. In our series, injection of saline between the mucosa and the posterior cyst wall helped us in successful excision by raising a plane of dissection (Figs. 5.34, 5.35, 5.36 & 5.37). The mucosal lining of the retained cyst wall should be ablated by diathermy, as 57% of the cholangiocarcinomas in a choledochal cyst arises from the posterior wall of the cyst[44]. It is important to note that fulguration is safe only if the posterior layer of the cyst is thick from chronic inflammation, otherwise, there is danger of thermal injury to underlying portal vein. The procedure was performed in 25 (48%) cases in our study owing to the same indications proposed by Lilly, while it was necessary in about 10% of the cases in one series[43]. Although it seems that the percentage of this procedure was large, but we believe that, intra- and postoperative complications in our study were quite less in patients undergoing Lilly's procedure.

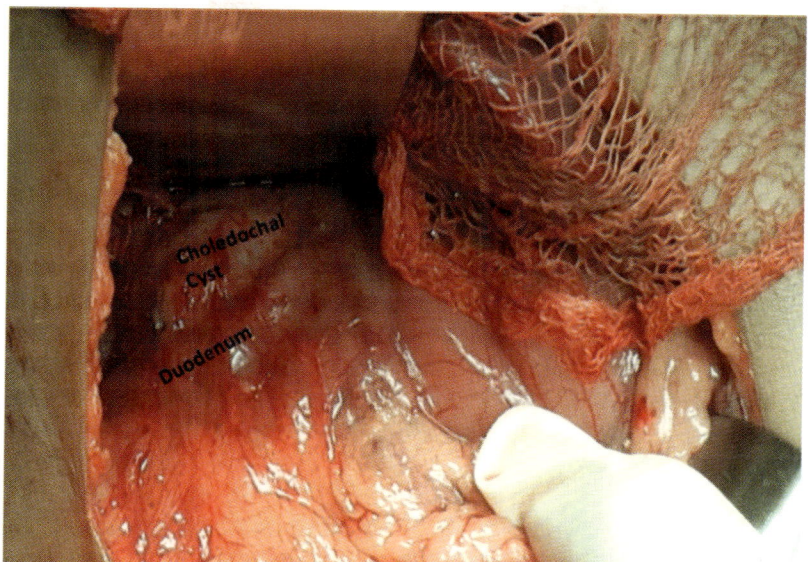

Fig. 5.32. Intraoperative photograph showing the classical variety of choledochal cyst (type IA). This patient had recurrent episodes of pancreatitis in the past. The cyst on exploration was found to be densely adherent to the duodenum and its posterior wall to the portal vein.

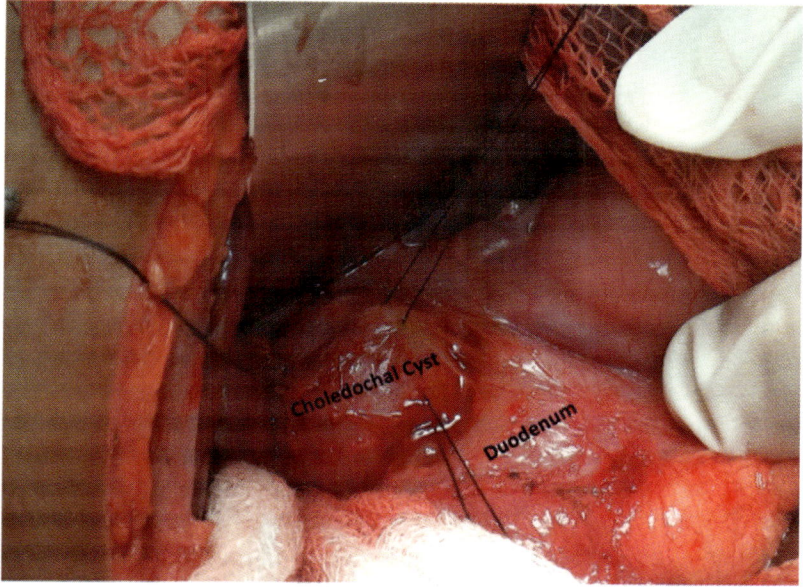

Fig. 5.33. Intraoperative photograph – stay sutures have been applied to the cyst wall and Lilly's procedure undertaken.

We care and he cures

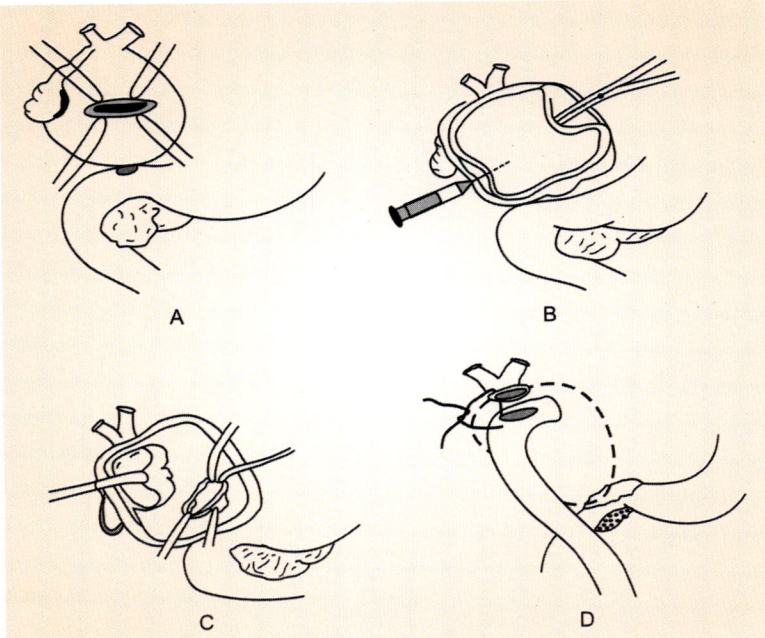

Fig. 5.34. Diagrammatic representation of steps followed for performing Lilly's procedure: Picture A: Stay sutures are applied to the cyst wall and cyst is opened with diathermy. Picture B: After excision of anterior and lateral walls of the cyst. A plane is created between the mucosa and remaining posterior wall of the cyst by injecting normal saline. Picture C: Removal of mucosal lining of the retained posterior wall of the cyst. Obliteration of duodenal end of the cyst. Picture D: End to side Roux-en-Y hepaticojejunostomy.

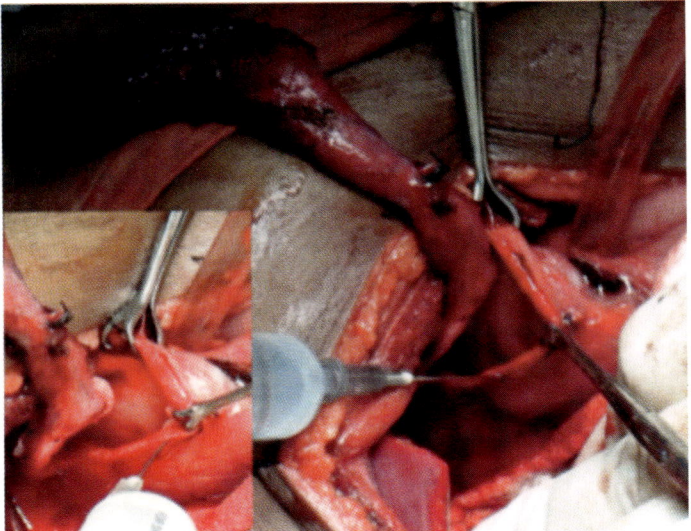

Fig. 5.35. Choledochal cyst opened anteriorly. Plane being created between mucosa and remaining posterior wall (Lilly's procedure) of cyst by injecting normal saline.

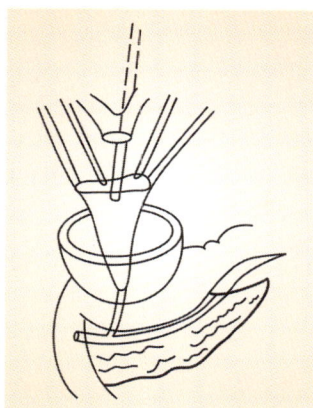

Fig. 5.36. Diagrammatic representation of Lilly's procedure. Mucosectomy with the help of stay sutures being performed from distal portion of cyst wall.

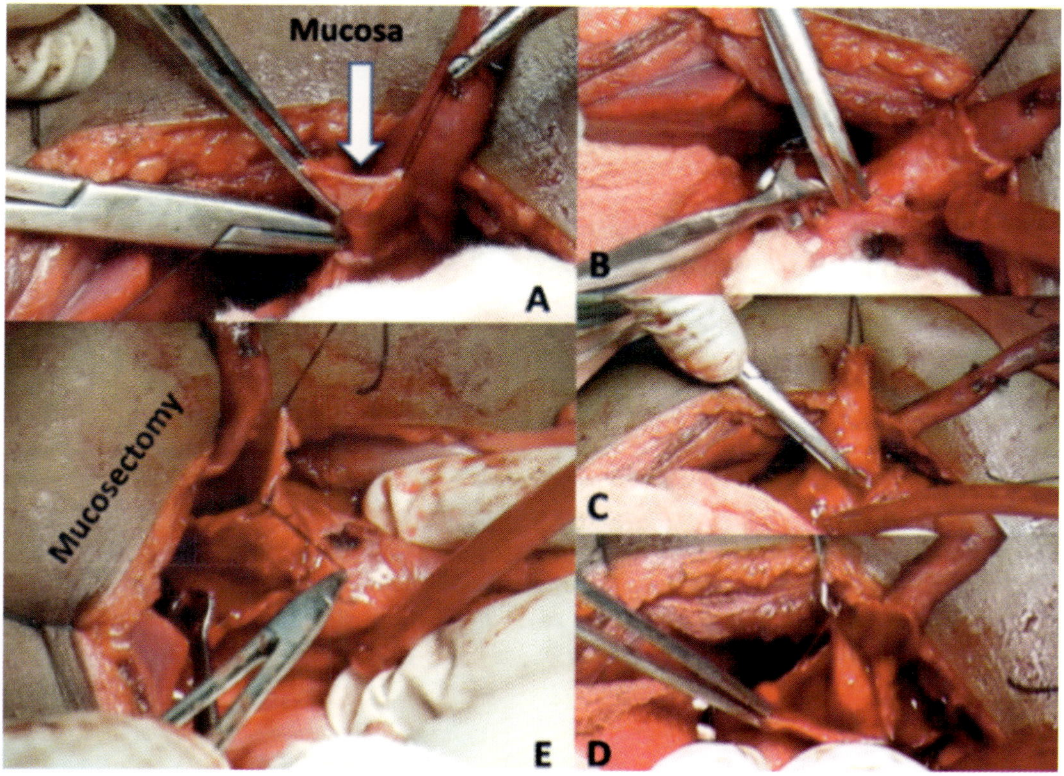

Fig. 5.37. Intraoperative photograph showing technique of Lilly's procedure. Plane of dissection is being created between mucosa and remaining posterior wall of cyst.

Child should not be treated as a miniature adult.

LAPAROSCOPIC EXCISION

Laparoscopic cyst excision and hepaticojejunostomy have been performed with principles similar to that of open surgery. It was first described by Farello et al. in 1995. Its limitation is small working space in small children and is technically demanding because of its close proximity to portal vein and hepatic artery, while the advantages are excellent visualization and magnification[45]. Moreover, a long subcostal incision is avoided with it. Proficiency in intracorporeal suturing and knotting is fundamental for secure and successful anastomosis[45]. It is reserved for experienced laparoscopic surgeons with an advanced laparoscopic training. A steep learning curve is present in the initial stage. There is a loss of direct hepatic feedback. Use of ultrasonic shears may be extremely useful for meticulous dissection.

STEPS OF LAPAROSCOPIC CYST EXCISION AND HEPATICOJEJUNOSTOMY

Patient is positioned in supine, catheterization and nasogastric tube is placed. Sand bag is placed under right hypochondrium. Pneumoperitoneum is created either with open Hasson technique or closed Veress needle technique through the umbilicus. During 1st blind insertion of trochar, child should be in 10–15 degrees Trendelenburg's position with direction of trochar towards the pelvis. The port position (Table 5.2) and team set-up is the same as the North American position for laparoscopic cholecystectomy except an extra 5-mm port for duodenal retraction is placed in the left lumbar area, along the left midclavicular line. Right hand working port may be placed to the left and higher of midline as shown in Fig. 5.38[45]. The left lobe of the liver is retracted cranially with a 5-mm grasper holding the gallbladder fundus. Additional ports are used for lifting quadrate lobe and for enough exposure of hilum. Abdomen is surfed to assess the status of the liver and to look for signs of portal hypertension. Adequate exposure of the working area is achieved by cranial retraction of the gallbladder and caudal traction of the transverse colon and duodenum. Steps of laparoscopic cyst excision and hepaticojejunostomy remain same as in open surgery[45]. The gallbladder is decompressed in case of gross distention. Kocherisation is performed with 15–20 degree left lateral tilt. Use of 3-mm short laparoscope is used in the paediatric population.

Number	Instrument	Place	Port size
1	Camera	Umbilicus	3.5/5/10 mm
2	Right hand working port	Epigastric	3.5/5 mm
3	Left hand working port	Right subcostal	3.5/5 mm
4	Gallbladder retracting port	Right lateral	3.5/5 mm
5	Duodenum retracting port	Left pararectus	3.5/5 mm

Table 5.2. Instrument and port positions

DISSECTION OF THE CYST

The peritoneum over the cyst just superior to the first part of the duodenum is incised and continued laterally up to the inferior vena cava. The inferior part of the cyst is then exposed by dissecting the superior and posterior parts of first part of the duodenum off the cyst. A careful assessment is done for malignancy, such as papillary projections, and vascular

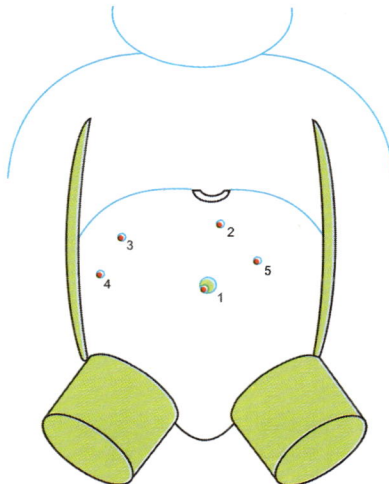

Fig. 5.38. Port positions in the patient for choledochal cyst excision.

involvement using laparoscopic ultrasonography (if available). If there is any suspicion of malignancy, conversion to laparotomy is done. The cyst is then decompressed by percutaneous aspiration and the bile sent for culture. Dissection is kept as close as possible to the wall without isolating the portal vein and the hepatic artery for preventing inadvertent injury. In the case of a large cyst, a transverse incision is made on the anterior wall and the debris and sludge evacuated. The transverse incision over the anterior wall is enlarged toward the left to dissect the medial cyst wall from the right hepatic artery with blunt dissection (suction nozzle). Separation of the posterior cyst wall from the portal vein may be performed by same technique. The posterior wall of the cyst is retracted with a grasper from the epigastric port to aid in this part of the dissection. In patients with recurrent attacks of cholangitis, Lilly's mucosectomy technique is carried out. Dissection is then extended cranially up to the level of the normal-sized hepatic ducts, and the cyst is completely excised along with gallbladder. The specimen should be placed in endobag and extracted through umbilical port. It is important to use gallbladder for retraction of the liver during the initial phase of the operation and perform cholecystectomy only at the end. This greatly enhances the vision in the hilar area for subsequent dissection.

In patients with smaller cysts, the entire cyst is mobilized circumferentially without decompression. The distal CBD is divided at its normal caliber, and is sutured with intracorporeal knotting. An attempt is ought to be made to demonstrate the junction of the choledochal cyst and the pancreatic duct in cases of APBDJ. In type IVA cysts, the proximal line of resection should ideally be extended up to the confluence of the right and left hepatic ducts.

ROUX-EN-Y LOOP CREATION

The duodenojejunal flexure is identified and the jejunum, at the level of the first good vascular arcade, is divided with an Endo-GIA linear cutter. 40 cm of the Roux limb is used for hepaticojejunostomy (30 cm in infants). The jejunojejunostomy is established at about

15–30 cm side-to-side intracorporeal anastomosis by intracorporeal knotting or using endo-staplers. The Roux loop is constructed entirely intracorporeally and brought up for the anastomosis in a retrocolic fashion, so that the long limb lay close to the lateral abdominal wall.

HEPATICOJEJUNOSTOMY

The hepaticojejunostomy is performed in an end-to-side fashion by intracorporeal suturing. For small ducts (< 1.5 cm) only, a cuff of proximal cyst is retained to aid in anastomosis. Also, a slit is made on one side of the duct so that the anastomosis lies in an oblique orientation, providing a wide lumen. An 18-French decompression tube may be placed at the level of the anastomosis and the end of the decompression tube is brought out through a small enterotomy made on the long limb of the Roux-en-Y loop that now lies more laterally. The enterotomy site is then fixed to the anterior abdominal wall by taking three or four intracorporeal sutures. The ports are closed after placement of a drain in the subhepatic space. Complications due to pneumoperitoneum especially in smaller children are gas embolism, cardiovascular compromise, and hypercapnia. Robotic approach has also been illustrated and seems to be as feasible as laparoscopy.

ALTERNATIVE PROCEDURES

HEPATICODUODENOSTOMY

Hepaticoduodenostomy has been proposed by some researchers to be more physiologically and technically easier, shorter operative time, and avoidance of intestinal anastomosis, fewer complications such as anastomotic leakage, postoperative adhesive bowel obstruction, and peptic ulcer and because there is delivery of bile into the duodenum, rather than into a Roux-en Y limb of the jejunum. There is ease of postoperative endoscopic evaluation. Its indication is when the lumen of duct is less than 1 cm in diameter after cyst excision. It involves duodenal mobilization to reach the porta hepatis without undue tension. Anastomosis is made with the duct at superoposterior part of the first part of duodenum. An abdominal drain is kept near the anastomosis as the reported incidence of leak is 10% with this procedure.

Intrahepatic biliary duct dilatation or when the diameter of the common hepatic duct is more than 10 mm is a contraindication, as duodenal contents are likely to reflux easily into the intrahepatic ducts through the anastomosis and its stasis causes bile duct mucosal damage, cholangitis or anastomotic stricture formation. Incidence of gastritis induced by duodeno-gastric bile reflux is high in patients with hepaticoduodenostomy. Although it is believed to be a safe and physiologic procedure, but it is not in practice.

JEJUNAL INTERPOSITION

The valved jejunal interposition hepaticoduodenostomy has been proposed by some surgeons has not gained much importance. Proximal jejunal interposition (30 cm isolated conduit), isoperistaltically or reversed segment between the confluence of hepatic duct and the duodenum. A single jejunal segment from the first or second jejunal loop is isolated. These are placed in retrocolic position to prevent reflux.

APPENDIX INTERPOSITION

It is also known as hepaticoappendicoduodenostomy. It is a method of using appendix with its vascularized pedicle as the conduit between hepatic ducts and duodenum. The caecum and the ascending colon up to the hepatic flexure are mobilized so that the appendix could lie next to the duodenum. The appendix is then divided at its base carefully while preserving the appendicular artery and mobilized for about 4–5 cm. The caecal defect is closed in two layers. The appendiceal graft patency is confirmed. The wider caecal end of the appendix is anastomosed to the common hepatic duct in an end-to-end manner. The appendiceal graft is then refashioned by excising the distal 2 cm to prevent kinking. The appendix is then anastomosed to the posterior aspect of the 2nd part of the duodenum in an end-to-side fashion.

The merits of using the appendix as a conduit are:

1. A vascularized patent conduit of small caliber, anatomically similar and excellent replacement for the native bile duct.
2. It avoids a long Roux loop with its associated complications of blind loop, stasis and need for intestinal anastomosis.
3. It is more physiological, as bile is drained into the duodenum in contrast to the Roux-en-Y limb.
4. A procedure with fewer suture lines.
5. Allows postoperative evaluation using endoscopic techniques.
6. Potential to decrease the incidence of postoperative cholangitis.

The demerit of using appendix as a conduit is that appendix graft undergoes stenosis, with subsequent biliary obstruction resulting in hepatic fibrosis. Owing to these reasons, this technique is not practised by the authors.

ABERRANT HEPATIC DUCT

Aberrant hepatic duct (AHD) is thought to be the result of normal variation in the development of the biliary system, and its incidence is as low as 5% in the normal population. It is not clinically important for the normal population, but it is a significant adjunct during surgery for choledochal cyst. An AHD may be connected with the main biliary system, or it may be a completely independent duct functioning to drain a portion of the bile flow. It may join the biliary tree at cystic duct, gallbladder, right hepatic duct, CBD or CHD. It is an extra-segmental or sub-segmental bile duct that often drains a part of the right hepatic lobe. It may be present in up to one-third of cases of choledochal cyst.

Knowledge of this entity is important for preventing damage to this structure and prevention of postoperative bile leak and further complications. Arbitrary ligation of the AHD independently responsible for drainage of part of the bile flow will obstruct the corresponding intrahepatic bile duct and result in such complications as liver cirrhosis and infection. In case of small AHD, its accidental ligation may result in atrophy of the obstructed segment. In large AHD options are re-establishment of the separate biliary enteric anastomosis with AHD, using appendix with its vascularized pedicle as the conduit between AHD and Roux-en-Y hepaticojejunostomy, and anastomosing AHD to main duct before performing Roux-en-Y hepaticojejunostomy. The last procedure has been recommended as a better technique by most series.

POSTOPERATIVE COMPLICATIONS

Complete excision with Roux-en-Y hepaticojejunostomy is the standard treatment with good surgical outcome for choledochal cyst. Postoperative morbidity with this procedure is 15–30%, mainly due to surgical wound infection, intra-abdominal sepsis, cholangitis and leakage of the anastomosis, which in most cases are managed conservatively[45, 46]. The complication rates are significantly lower in children as compared to adults. Surgical wound and postoperative scars are shown in Figs. 5.39, 5.40 & 5.41.

Incidence of postoperative biliary leak is reduced by wide-caliber hepaticojejunostomy, and to the normal bile duct, using a meticulous surgical technique to avoid leaks. Other complications include ileus, gastrointestinal bleeding, and bowel perforation. In our study, there was no postoperative haematoma or subhepatic collection, as seen in another study[8, 43]. In our study total postoperative complications were seen in 15 (28.8%) patients[8].

Postoperative pancreatitis with or without protein plug is rare after cyst excision and internal drainage. Rarely, patients may develop pancreatitis after cyst excision and internal

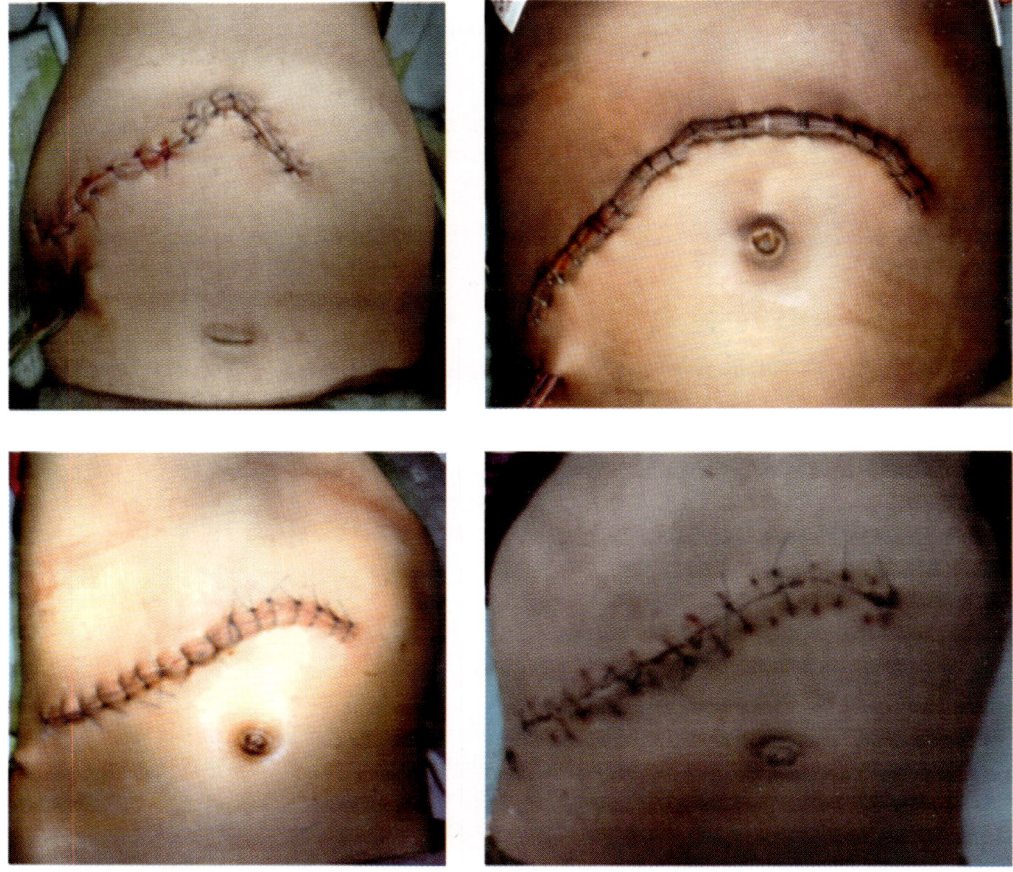

Fig. 5.39. Sutured wound (roof-top/cheveron incision) of choledochal cyst in postoperative period (in different patients).

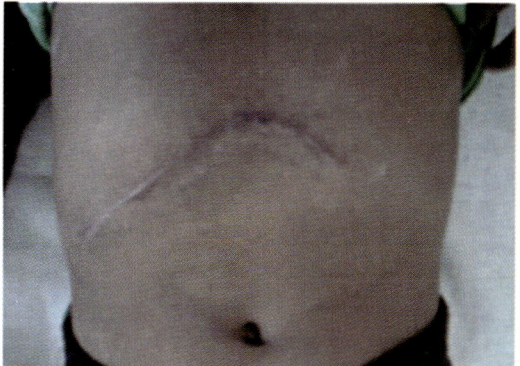

Fig. 5.40. Ideal postoperative scar of cheveron incision, with left limb smaller than the right limb.

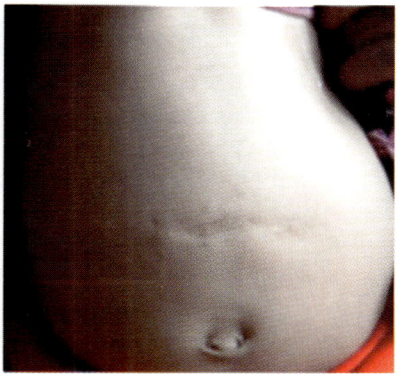

Fig. 5.41. Postoperative scar in other patient.

drainage. The morphology of pancreatic duct and its dilatation, possibly caused by stasis of pancreatic juice, or residual abnormalities of common channel may be the etiological factors[27].

Cholangitis is a common complication after surgical management. For prevention of cholangitis, broad-spectrum antibiotic therapy directed against common biliary pathogens, such as *Escherichia coli* and *Klebsiella* species, in addition to other supportive measures.

Postoperative anastomotic strictures have been proposed by Japanese to be related to severity of mucosal denudation of CHD, intramural fibrosis, ischemia or prolonged inflammation secondary to bile stasis in intrahepatic biliary tree. Anastomotic strictures are associated with intrahepatic cholelithiasis and cholangitis. It is reduced by performing a higher anastomosis, i.e. hepaticojejunostomy rather than choledochojejunostomy[47]. Intraoperative use of endoscopy to carefully determine the level of resection of CHD is advocated by Japanese group. Also, Japanese group recommends hepaticojejunostomy at the hepatic hilum to create a wide stoma by incising along the lateral walls of the hepatic duct (Fig. 5.24) following excision of the narrowed segment of CHD (which may be chronically inflamed and fibrotic).

Reoperation for recurrent cholangitis secondary to stenosis has been reported to be from 13% to 69%[48]. A wide anastomosis aims to prevent persistent cholestasis which may be a high-risk factor for carcinogenesis[48]. Roux-en-Y limb stomas and Hutson access limbs have been used to facilitate endoscopic access to anastomotic strictures. Reoperation for revision of hepaticojejunostomy is the most common and important indication. Other indications for reoperation are biliary lithiasis, endoscopic sphincterotomy of the ampulla of Vater, adhesion obstruction, pancreaticojejunostomy and lobectomy.

Roux syndrome is the main complication of Roux-en-Y procedure. This syndrome consists of chronic abdominal pain, nausea, and vomiting that are worsened by eating. It may worsen either by eating either solids or liquids. These patients are frequently considered as having psychosomatic disease. It is secondary to gastric or efferent jejunal stasis, or both. Treatment involves round the clock analgesics and prokinetics.

Intrahepatic stones/lithiasis are a particular problem in cases of type IV disease with residual intrahepatic cysts and in type V. Predisposing factors are preexisting stricture or ductal obstruction (as in type V) leading to bile stasis, which plays an important role in its pathogenesis. Choledocholithiasis, intrapancreatic terminal choledochus calculi, pancreatic ductal calculi have been reported. This complication has been reported to be lower in patients who undergo intraoperative choledochoscopy/endoscopy. The complications may be related to residual terminal cyst and APBDJ. Choledochoscopy and intraoperative cholangiography with ductal probing and washout of debris reduces postoperative complications of stones retained in the biliary radicals. The stone formation is more in adults as compared to paediatric patients. Calculus in the residual portion of the intrapancreatic cyst has been reported to cause relapsing pancreatitis. Also, stone in the blind pouch of an end to side hepaticojejuno-stomy has been described in the literature. Intracystic lithiasis is frequently associated with tumour, and can give similar radiological appearances[49]. Ursodeoxycholic acid may improve bile flow, reducing the incidence of biliary sludge, stones, and cholangitis.

Intestinal obstruction due to adhesions and internal herniae of the small bowel is a recognised complication of Roux-en-Y bypass procedures[34]. Biliary stasis secondary to anastomotic stricture and bowel obstruction may be related to elongation of the blind pouch (from end-to-side anastomosis) or redundant Roux jejunal limb as they have the potential to grow or elongate in children.

Intrahepatic bile duct dilatation has been associated with late postoperative complications if associated with downstream stenosis. In adult patients, wall of intrahepatic bile ducts may be severely and irreversibly damaged resulting in poor resolution of involved intrahepatic bile duct dilatation. Various procedures recommended intraoperatively in the literature are intrahepatic ductoplasty, intrahepatic cystojejunostomy, balloon dilatation of the stenosis, hepaticojejunostomy at the hepatic hilum to create a wide stoma and segmentectomy of the liver. In our experience with paediatric patients, intrahepatic bile duct dilatation resolved with definitive surgery and we believe it to be a cause and effect relationship.

MALIGNANT CHANGE AFTER CYST EXCISION

The risk of post-excision malignancy increases with age, rising from 0.7% in patients with cysts operated upto 10 years of age, to 6.6% when operated between 11–20 years, and 14.3% if first treated at > 20 years old[50]. It is more common in cysts of Alonso-Lej types I, IV and V[49]. Todani et al. observed 68% of malignancy in type I, 5% in type II, 1.6% in type III, 21% in type IV, and 6% in type V[47]. Malignancy in choledochal cyst occurs more commonly in cysts and in "Forme Fruste" at the gallbladder. Malignancy in Caroli's disease is reported to be about 7–15% and in choledochoceles about 2.5%. Malignancy occurs in 12–39% of "Forme Fruste" patients.

It is postulated that it can occur in residual intrapancreatic portion of the choledochal cyst, in cases with intrapancreatic extension, and in most of the cases, the cause may be attributed to incomplete resection[51]. Its excision is recommended for its prevention. Postoperative stenosis and repeated cholangitis lead to bile stasis and intrahepatic lithiasis which may be a high-risk factor for carcinogenesis[52]. Malignancy in patients with incomplete cyst resection is high as compared with complete cyst resection. Malignancy has been reported to arise in the intrahepatic cysts, intrahepatic bile duct or residual common bile duct following resection of the cyst, terminal CBD and HJ anastomotic site[51–55]. In our series out of 52 cases, including 25 (48%) who underwent Lilly's procedure, none of the patients had malignant transformation of the residual cyst wall and same holds good for 75 patients, including 10% cases who underwent Lilly's procedure in one large series[8, 43]. It is believed that duration of chronic inflammation is expected to be shorter in children and the occurrence of malignancy in children is less as compared to adults[33–35].

POSTOPERATIVE FOLLOW-UP

To protect against the cholangitis, we keep the patients on low doses of antibiotics for approximately 6 weeks postoperatively. During this period, patient is rigorously assessed clinically for any features of cholangitis. The potential for this complication decreases after this period. Incidence of postoperative cholangitis is less as compared to biliary atresia. Choleretics like ursodeoxycholic acid can decrease bile viscosity and facilitate the drainage of bile, thereby improving bile passage. Three monthly follow-ups for the first year and annually thereafter is recommended. Liver function studies and serum amylase levels are carried at each visit. Annual ultrasound of the liver and pancreas is done, particularly in those having intrahepatic ductal dilatation preoperatively or when symptomatic (Figs. 5.42, 5.43, 5.44 and 5.45). It is an extremely useful investigation for identifying the postoperative complications. DISIDA scanning together with ultrasonography is very helpful for post-

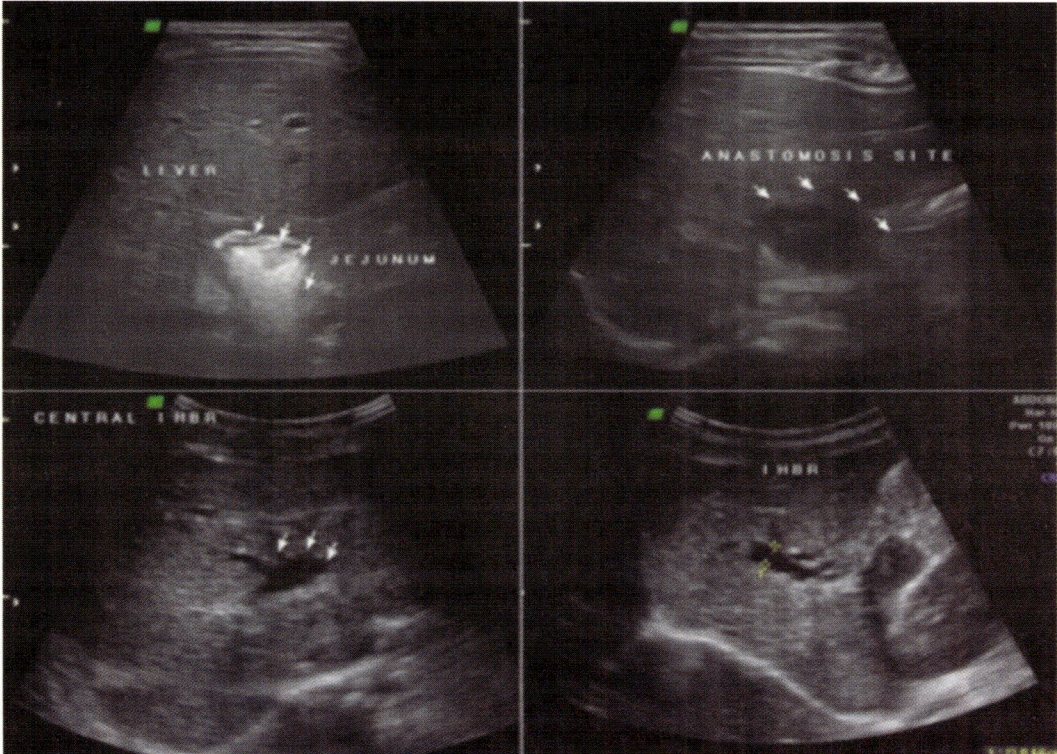

Fig. 5.42. Ultrasound images of postoperative case of type IVA patient showing the HJ (hepaticojejunostomy) anastomotic site. There is minimal dilatation of IHBR (Intra Hepatic Biliary Radicals) postoperatively (hence a cause and effect relationship). Kindly compare it with Fig. 4.3.

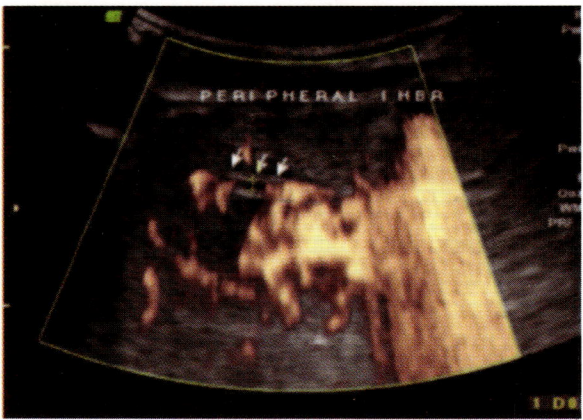

Fig. 5.43. Colour Doppler ultrasound image showing resolution of cystic dilatation of IHBR with normal vascular flow in type IVA choledochal cyst.

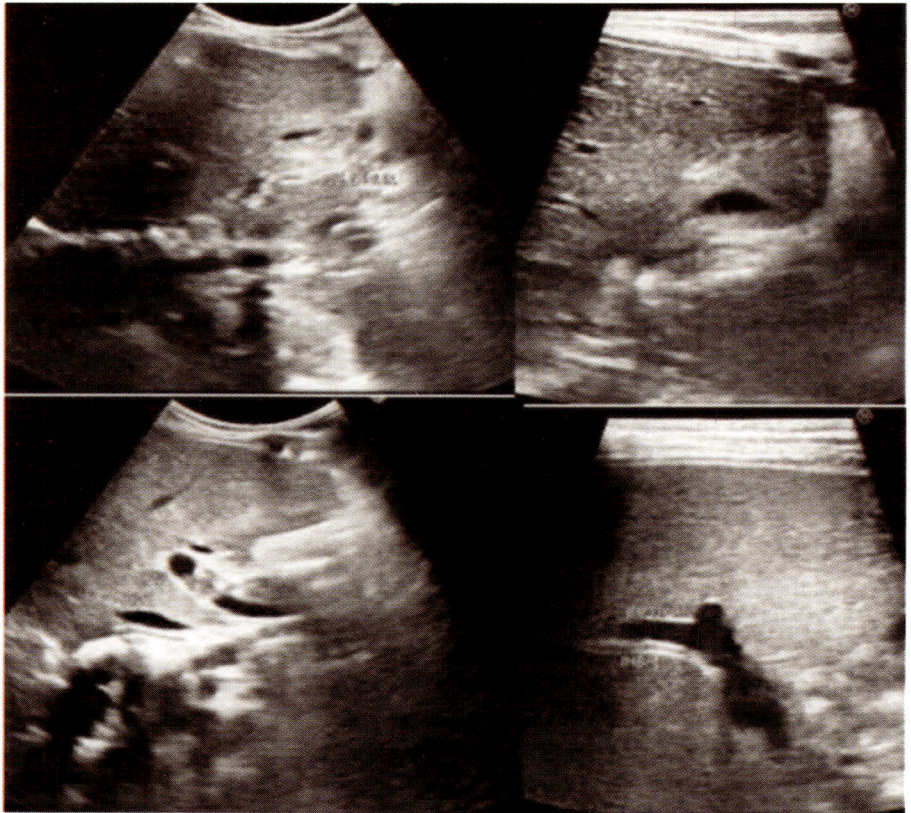

Fig. 5.44. Postoperative ultrasound of type IA patient showing the HJ (hepaticojejunostomy) anastomotic site in upper images. There is absence of dilatation of IHBR (Intra Hepatic Biliary Radicals) postoperatively as shown in lower images. Portal vein is seen in close relationship to IHBR.

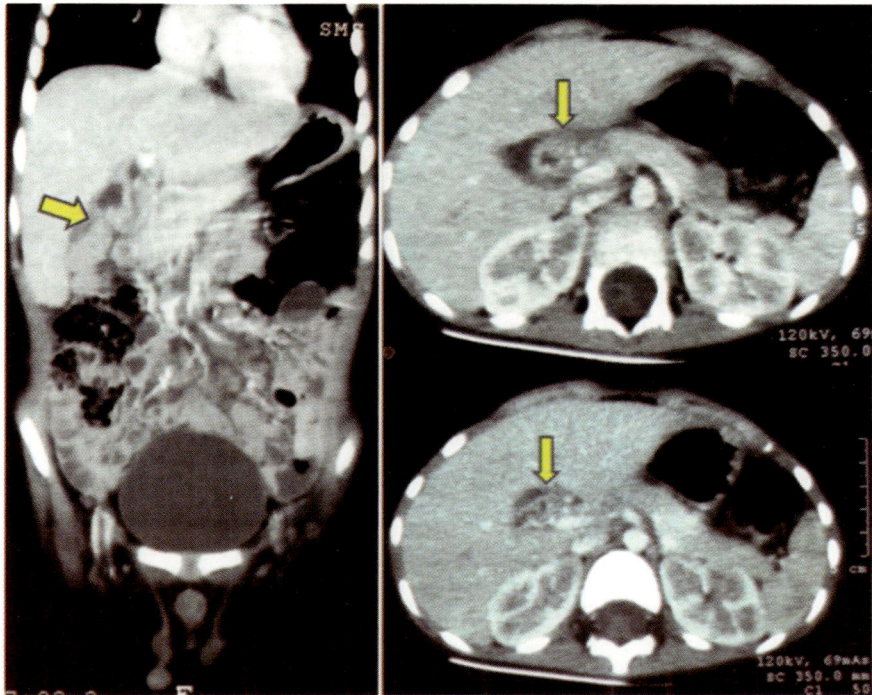

Fig. 5.45. Postoperative CECT images of type IA patient showing the HJ (hepaticojejunostomy) anastomotic site, with Roux limb (yellow arrow). There is absence of dilatation of IHBR (Intra Hepatic Biliary Radicals).

operative follow-up examinations (Figs. 5.46 & 5.47). MRCP permits safe serial screening for malignant complications in the postoperative years. ERCP is often difficult after Roux-en-Y hepaticojejunostomy.

Long-term surveillance is crucial in patients, especially if there was dilatation of the intrahepatic bile duct, dilatation of the remaining distal bile duct, pancreatic duct, APBDJ or biliary stones. Other important considerations are rate of bile excretion, any degree of stasis, sludge or stones. Patient, who underwent endoscopic sphincterotomy for choledochocele, should undergo endoscopic surveillance since malignancy has been reported in choledochocele. Postoperative evolution will be satisfactory if biliary flow is adequate with symptom resolution in > 80% of cases[7].

PROGNOSIS

Choledochal cyst generally shows an excellent long-term prognosis with early resectional surgery and Roux-en-Y hepaticojejunostomy. Good prognosis is expected in patients who undergo complete resection of cyst and biliary diversion after previous cystenterostomy.

In patients with postoperative biliary dysfunction after cyst internal drainage, there is strong indication for revision with cyst excision. Untreated choledochal cysts uniformly have poor prognoses. Poorer prognosis is related to patients who presented with serious deterioration of the hepatic function at diagnosis, late presentation with cirrhosis, portal

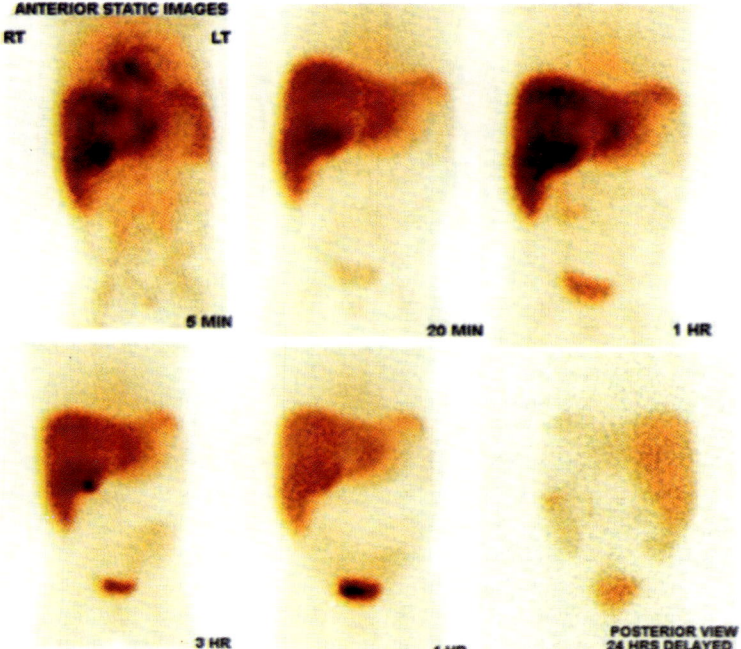

Fig. 5.46. Tc-99m HIDA (hepatobiliary scintigram) three months postoperatively showing absence of free flow of radiopharmaceutical into the bowel in one of our patients. This patient had secondary biliary cirrhosis preoperatively.

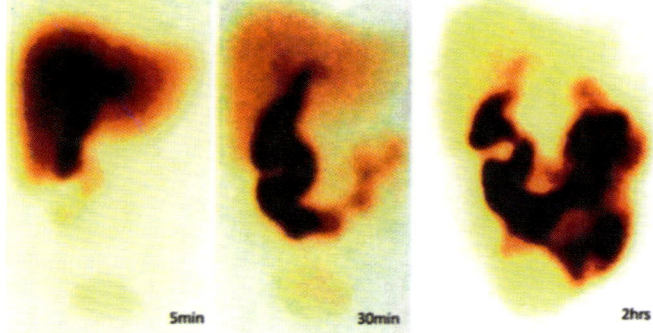

Fig. 5.47. Tc-99m HIDA scan. Static images were taken in anterior projection after i.v. injection of Tc-99m Mebrofenin, showing normal liver function and unobstructed biliary drainage into the bowel. The indication for performing scan was pain abdomen postoperatively, when all other investigations were normal.

hypertension, associated pancreatitis, and superadded infection. Malignant transformation is the most serious complication, usually seen in adults with a poor prognosis. Patients with intraoperative findings of malignancy, survival rate is low.

Adult form has better prognosis than infantile form. On the other hand infantile form of choledochal cyst has good prognosis as compared to biliary atresia, despite the presence of bridging fibrosis and cirrhosis in some cases[56].

SURGICAL CLASSIFICATION

We believe classification into type I to type V and further sub-classification of type I into A, B and C according to Todani's classification does not have much influence on the surgical management and outcome[8]. Surgical management for type IA, type IB, type IC, type II and type IVB is complete excision of the involved portion of the extrahepatic bile duct from the hepatic hilum to the pancreaticobiliary duct junction with Roux-en-Y hepaticojejunostomy[40]. Also for type IVA initial surgical management is same, as intrahepatic duct dilatation is a cause and effect relationship (Figs. 5.42 & 5.43)[8, 41, 57]. Resection of the affected hepatic segment or lobe is indicated in case of complications as discussed earlier. Management for type III is mainly endoscopic, unless it is larger than 3 cm or there is duodenal obstruction.

We propose and classify choledochal cyst into:

- Type R (Roux-en-Y): Cases requiring Roux-en-Y hepaticojejunostomy – Type IA, Type IB, Type IC, Type II, Type IV A and Type IV B of Todani's classification.
- Type E (Endoscopic): Cases requiring endoscopic management – Type III of Todani's classification.
- Type V is entirely an intrahepatic disease and there is no extrahepatic dilatation of biliary tree as per the definition. The choledochus is normal and therefore it is an entirely different entity, requiring liver resections and transplantation.

CONCLUSION

Choledochal cyst present nonspecifically rather than classically. It requires proper diagnosis and treatment to address associated symptoms, risk of malignancy, and disease progression. A high index of suspicion will avoid a delay in diagnosis, especially while evaluating neonates and infants with cholestatic jaundice and older children with recurrent abdominal pain. The imaging modality of choice for diagnosing and characterizing choledochal cysts is, however, MRCP, but in our resource-limited set-up, it is an extremely difficult endeavour. We consider CECT as investigation of choice in smaller children.

Although the gold standard treatment for choledochal cyst is complete excision of the extrahepatic duct, cholecystectomy, and Roux-en-Y hepaticojejunostomy, but removal of adherent cyst wall to portal vein had no added benefit, rather it increased the morbidity in terms of intraoperative blood loss and postoperative complications. We believe and lay equal emphasis towards Lilly's procedure in cases with cyst densely adherent to the portal vein secondary to long-standing inflammation because of low surgical morbidity and mortality associated with it. Moreover, we didn't have any case of cholangiocarcinoma in our study. Long-term surveillance is essential to detect complications, such as cholangitis, anastomotic stricture, intrahepatic cholelithiasis and cholangiocarcinoma.

Not taking a correct history and not doing a thorough examination by inspection, palpation and auscultation can mislead the physician in achieving the goal. Therefore, a practitioner keen to carry out any procedure should first of all examine and thoroughly investigate the same before venturing on the case.

Sushruta

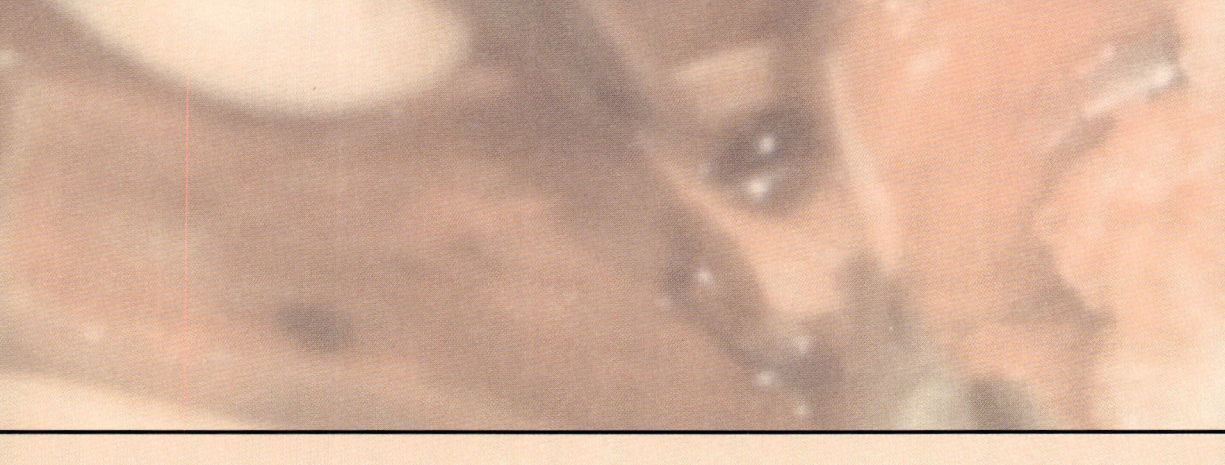

References

1. Saxena R, Pradeep R, Chander J, Kumar P, Wig JD, Yadav RV, Kaushik SP. Benign disease of the common bile duct. *Br J Surg*, 1988; 75 (8): 803–6.
2. O'Neill JA, Templeton JM Jr, Schnaufer L, Bishop HC, Ziegler MM, Ross AJ 3rd. Recent experience with choledochal cyst. *Ann Surg*, 1987; 205: 533–40.
3. Gigot J, Nagorney D, Farnell M, Moir C, Ilstrup D. Bile duct cysts: A changing spectrum of disease. *J Hepatobiliary Pancreat Surg*, 1996; 3: 405–11.
4. Uribarrena Amezaga R, Raventos N, Fuentes J, Elias J, Tejedo V, Uribarrena Echebarria R. Diagnosis and management of choledochal cyst. A review of 10 new cases. *Rev Esp Enferm Dig*, 2008; 10: 71–5.
5. Skapinker S. Choledochal Cyst. *S.A. Medical Journal*, 1956; 2: 403.
6. Alonso-Lej F, Rever WB Jr, Pessagno DJ. Congenital choledochal cyst, with a report of 2, and an analysis of 94, cases. *Int Abstr Surg*, 1959; 108: 1–30.
7. Todani T, Watanabe Y, Narusue M, Tabuchi K, Okajima K. Congenital bile duct cysts: Classification, operative procedures, and review of thirty-seven cases including cancer arising from choledochal cyst. *Am J Surg*, 1977; 134: 263–9.
8. Gupta R, Sharma SB, Soni V, Mathur P. Management dilemma with choledochal cyst in paediatric patients: a single institution experience. *CIBTech Journal of Surgery*, 2014; 3 (1): 27–37.
9. Kim OH, Chung HJ, Choi BG. Imaging of the choledochal cyst. *Radiographics*, 1995; 15 (1): 69–88.
10. Miyano T, Li L, Yamataka A. Choledochal cyst. *In* Textbook of Pediatric Surgery – Diagnosis and Management, Vol 2, Section: 5 (Hepatobiliary System): 1013–25.
11. Hung MH, Lin LH, Chen DF, Huang CS. Choledochal cyst in infants and children: experiences over a 20-year period at a single institution. *Eur J Pediatr*, 2011; 170: 1179–85.

12. Singham J, Schaeffer D, Yoshida E, Scudamore C. Choledochal cysts: analysis of disease pattern and optimal treatment in adult and paediatric patients. *HPB*, 2007; 9 (5): 383–7.
13. Linder HM, Green RB. Embryologic and surgical anatomy of the extra-hepatic biliary tree. *Surg Clin North Am*, 1964; 44: 1273–85.
14. Babbitt's DP. Congenital choledochal cyst: new etiological concept based on anomalous relationships of the common bile duct and pancreatic bulb. *Ann Radiol*, 1969; 12: 231–40.
15. Miyano T, Yamataka A. Choledochal cysts. *Curr Opin Pediatr*, 1997; 9 (3): 283–8.
16. Schweizer P, Schweizer M. Pancreaticobiliary long common channel syndrome and congenital anomalous dilatation of the choledochal duct: study of 46 patients. *Eur J Pediatr Surg*, 1993; 315–21.
17. Kusunoki M, Saitoh N, Yamamura T, Fujita S, Takahashi T, Utsunomiya J. Choledochal cysts: oligoganglionosis in the narrow portion of the choledochus. *Arch Surg*, 1988; 123: 984–986.
18. Kagiyama S, Okazaki K, Yamamoto Y, Yamamoto Y. Anatomic variants of choledocho-cele and manometric measurements of pressure in the cele and the orifice zone. *Am J Gastroenterol*, 1987; 82: 641–9.
19. Landing BH. Considerations of the pathogenesis of neonatal hepatitis, biliary atresia and choledochal cyst: the concept of infantile obstructive cholangiopathy. *Prog Pediatr Surg*, 1974; 6: 113–39.
20. Tyler KL, Sokol RJ, Oberhaus SM, Le M, Karrer FM, Narkewicz MR, Tyson RW, Murphy JR, Low R, Brown WR. Detection of reovirus RNA in hepatobiliary tissues from patients with extrahepatic biliary atresia and choledochal cysts. *Hepatology*, 1998; 27 (6): 1475–82.
21. Douglas AH. Case of dilatation of the common bile duct. *Monthly J Med Sci*, 1852; 14: 97–101.
22. Watanatittan S, Niramis R. Choledochal cyst: review of 74 pediatric cases. *J Med Assoc Thai*, 1998; 81: 586–95.
23. Stringer MD, Dhawan A, Davenport M, Mieli-Vergani G, Mowat AP, Howard ER. Choledochal cysts: lessons from a 20 year experience. *Arch Dis Child*, 1995; 73: 528–31.
24. Samuel M, Spitz L. Choledochal cyst: varied clinical presentations and long-term results of surgery. *Eur J Pediatr Surg*, 1996; 678–81.
25. Lipsett PA, Pitt HA, Colombani PM, Boitnott JK, Cameron JL. Choledochal cyst disease: a changing pattern of presentation. *Ann Surg*, 1994; 220: 644–52.
26. Dudin A, Abdelshafi M, Cousson AR. Choledochal cyst associated with rare hand malformation. *American Journal of Medical Genetics*, 1995; 56: 161–3.
27. Swisher SG, Cates JA, Hunt KK, Robert ME, Bennion RS, Thompson JE, et al. Pancreatitis associated with adult choledochal cysts. *Pancreas*, 1994; 9: 633–7.
28. Nambirajan L, Taneja P, Singh MK, Mitra DK, Bhatnagar V. The liver in choledochal cyst. *Trop Gastroenterol*, 2000; 21: 135–9.
29. Saluja SS, Mishra PK, Sharma BC, Narang P. Management of choledochal cyst with portal hypertension. *Singapore Med J*, 2011; 52 (12): e239.
30. Yeong ML, Nicholson GI, Lee SP. Regression of biliary cirrhosis following choledochal cyst drainage. *Gastroenterology*, 1982; 82: 332–5.

31. Iwai N, Deguchi E, Yanagihara J, Iwai M, Matsuo H, Todo S, Imashuku S. Cancer arising in a choledochal cyst in a 12-year-old girl. *J Pediatr Surg*, 1990; 25 (12): 1261–3.

32. Rattner DW, Schapiro RH, Warshaw AL. Abnormalities of the pancreatic and biliary ducts in adult patients with choledochal cysts. *Arch Surg*, 1983; 118: 1068–73.

33. Bismuth H, Krissat J. Choledochal cystic malignancies. *Ann Oncol*, 1999; 10: 94–8.

34. Ong J, Campbell W, Taylor MA. Metastatic cholangiocarcinoma following choledochal cyst excision: an unusual cause of abdominal pain in a 35-year-old female. *Ulster Med J*, 2013; 82 (1): 21–2.

35. Song KH, Kim MH, Myung SJ, Lee SK, Kim HJ, Yoo KS, Seo DW, Lee HJ, Lim BC, Min YI. Choledochal cyst associated with the anomalous union of pancreaticobiliary duct (AUPBD) has a more grave clinical course than choledochal cyst alone. *Korean J Intern Med*, 1999; 14: 1–8.

36. Fieber SS, Nance FC. Choledochal cyst and neoplasm: a comprehensive review of 106 cases and presentation of two original cases. *Am Surg*, 1997; 63: 982–5.

37. Matsubara H, Oya N, Suzuki Y, Kajiura S, Suzumori K, Matsuo Y et al. Is it possible to differentiate between choledochal cyst and congenital biliary atresia (type I cyst) by antenatal ultrasonography? *Fetal Diagn Ther*, 1997; 12: 306–8.

38. Kim SH, Lim JH, Yoon HK, Han BK, Lee SK, Kim YI. Choledochal cyst: comparison of MR and conventional cholangiography. *Clin Radiol*, 2000; 55: 378–83.

39. Rosenfield N, Griscom NT. Choledochal cysts: roentgenographic techniques. *Radiology*, 1975; 114: 113–9.

40. Scudamore CH, Hemming AW, Teare JP, Fache JS, Erb SR, Watkinson AF. Surgical management of choledochal cysts. *Am J Surg*, 1994; 167: 497–500.

41. Hill R, Parsons C, Farrant P, Sellars M, Davenport M. Intrahepatic duct dilatation in type 4 choledochal malformation: pressure related, postoperative resolution. *J Pediatr Surg*, 2011; 46: 299–303.

42. Lilly JR. The surgical treatment of choledochal cyst. *Surg Gynecol Obstet*, 1979; 149: 36–42.

43. Lee KH, Tam YH, Chan EKW, Sihoe JDY, Cheung GST, Mou JWC. A Twenty-year Experience in Choledochal Cysts in Children: From Open to Laparoscopic Excision. *HK J Paediatr*, 2009; 14: 158–167.

44. Flanigan DP. Biliary carcinoma associated with biliary cysts. *Cancer*, 1977; 40: 880–3.

45. Palanivelu C, Rangarajan M, Parthasarathi R, Amar V, Senthilnathan P. Laparoscopic Management of Choledochal Cysts: Technique and Outcomes – A Retrospective Study of 35 Patients from a Tertiary Center. *J Am Coll Surg*, 2008; 207: 839–46.

46. Visser BC, Suh I, Way LW, Kang SM. Congenital choledochal cysts in adults. *Arch Surg*, 2004; 139: 855–60.

47. Todani T, Watanabe Y, Toki A, Ogura K, Wang ZQ. Co-existing biliary anomalies and anatomical variants in choledochal cyst. *Br J Surg*, 1998; 85: 760–3.

48. Chaudhari A, Dhar P, Sachdev A. Reoperative surgery for choledochal cysts. *Br J Surg*, 1997; 84: 781–4.

49. Dayton MT, Longmire WP Jr, Tompkins RK Caroli's Disease: A premalignant condition? *Am J Surg*, 1983; 145 (l): 41–8.

50. Voyles CR, Smajda C, Shand C Blumgart LH. Carcinoma in choledochal cysts-age related incidence. *Archives of Surgery*, 1983; 118: 986–8.
51. Watanabe Y, Toki A, Todani T. Bile duct cancer developed after cyst excision for choledochal cyst. *J Hepatobiliary Pancreat Surg*, 1999; 6: 207–12.
52. Ando H, Kaneko K, Ito T, Watanabe Y, Seo T, Harada T. Complete excision of the intrapancreatic portion of choledochal cysts. *J Am Coll Surg*, 1996; 183: 317–21.
53. Ono S, Sakai K, Kimura O, Iwai N. Development of bile duct cancer in a 26-year-old man after resection of infantile choledochal cyst. *J Pediatr Surg*, 2008; 43 (6): E17–9.
54. Miyano T, Yamataka A, Kato Y, Segawa O, Lane G, Takamizawa S, et al. Hepatico-enterostomy after excision of choledochal cyst in children: a 30 year experience with 180 cases. *J Paediatr Surg*, 1996; 31: 1417–21.
55. Miyano T, Yamataka A, Li L. Congenital biliary dilatation. *Semin Pediatr Surg*, 2000; 9: 187–95.
56. Vijayaraghavan P, Lal R, Sikora SS, Poddar U, Yachha SK. Experience with choledochal cysts in infants. *Pediatr Surg Int*, 2006; 22: 803–7.
57. Ohi R, Yaoita S, Kamiyama T, Ibrahim M, Hayashi Y, Chiba T. Surgical treatment of congenital dilatation of the bile duct with special reference to late complications after total excisional operation. *J Pediatr Surg*, 1990; 25: 613–7.

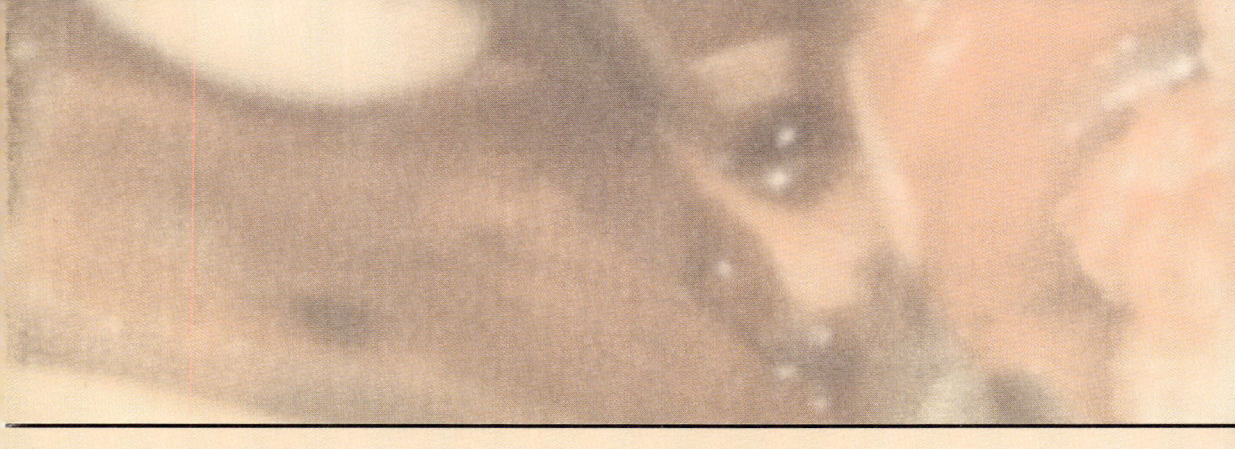

Further Reading

1. O'Neill JA (Junior). Chapter on *Choledochal Cyst*. Grosfeld JL, O'Neill JA (Junior), Fonkalsrud EW, Coran AG. **Paeditric Surgery**, 6th edition, Vol. 1, Mosby-Elsevier publications. 1620–34.
2. Clifton MS, Goldstein RB, Slavotinek A, Norton ME, Lee H, Farrell J, et al. Prenatal Diagnosis of Familial Type I Choledochal Cyst, *Pediatrics*, 2006; 117; e596–600.
3. Büyükyavuz Ý, Ekinci S, Çiftçi AÖ, Karnak Ý, Mehmet Emin, Þenocak, Tanyel FC, Büyükpamukçu N. A retrospective study of choledochal cyst: clinical presentation, diagnosis and treatment. *Turk J Pediatr*, 2003; 45: 321–325.
4. Bhavsar MS, Vora HB, Giriyappa VH. Choledochal cysts: A review of literature. *Saudi J Gastroenterol*, 2012; 18: 230–6.
5. The Japanese Study Group on Pancreaticobiliary Maljunction (JSPBM). The Committee of JSPBM for Diagnostic Criteria. Diagnostic criteria of pancreaticobiliary maljunction. *J Hepatobiliary Pancreat Surg*, 1994; 1: 219–21.
6. Greenholz SK, Lilly JR, Shikes RH, et al. Biliary atresia in the new-born. *J Pediatr S*, 1986; 21: 1147–8.
7. Choi KK, Choi SB, Park SW, Kim HK, Park YN, Kim KS. Synchronous double primary cancers associated with a choledochal cyst and anomalous pancreaticobiliary ductal union. *J Korean Surg Soc*, 2011; 81: 281–6.
8. Farello GA, Cerofolini A, Rebonato M, et al. Congenital Choledochal cyst: video-guided laparoscopic treatment. *Surg Laparosc Endosc*, 1995; 5: 354–8.
9. Takehara Y, Ichijo K, Tooyama N, Kodaira N, Yamamoto H, Totami M, Saito M, Watahiki H, Takahashi M. Breath-hold MR cholangiopancreatography with a long-echo-train fast spin-echo sequence and a surface coil in chronic pancreatitis. *Radiology*, 1994; 192: 73–78.
10. Matos C, Nicaise N, Deviere J, Cassart M, Metens T, Struyven J, Cremer M. Choledochal cysts: comparison of findings at MR cholangiopancreatography and endoscopic retrograde cholangiopancreatography in eight patients. *Radiology*, 1998; 209: 443–448.

11. Lam WW, Lam TP, Saing H, Chan FL, Chan KL. MR cholangiography and CT cholangiography of pediatric patients with choledochal cysts. *Am J Roentgenol*, 1999; 173: 401–405.

12. Lee MY, Juan CJ, Fan HC, Chao HM, Chu CC, Yuh YS et al. Choledochal Cysts in Children: A Case Report. *J M Med Sci*, 2002; 22 (2): 87–90.

13. Jaw TS, Huang BL, Wu CC. Ultrasonography and 99mTc-DISIDA cholescintigraphy in the diagnosis of choledochal cyst in children. *Kaohsiung J Med Sci*, 1989; 5: 688–696.

14. Ozawa K, Yamada T, Matsumoto Y, Tobe R (1980) Carcinoma arising in a choledochocele. *Cancer*, 45: 195–197.

15. Manning PB, Polley TZ, Jr., and Oldham KT. Choledochocele: an unusual form of choledochal cyst. *Pediatr Surg Int*, 1990; 5: 22–26.

16. Sawyer M, Katz J. Choledochal cysts. 2009; http://emedicine.medscape.com/article/172099.

17. Shah OJ, Shera AH, Zarger SA, Shah P, Robbani I, Dhar S, et al. Choledochal cysts in children and adults with contrasting profiles: 11 year experience at a training care center in Kashmir. *World J Surg*, 2009; 33 (11): 2403–11.

18. Funabiki T, Matsubara T, Miyakawa S, et al. Pancreaticobiliary maljunction and carcinogenesis to biliary and pancreatic malignancy. *Langenbeck's archives of surgery/Deutsche Gesellschaft fur Chirurgie*, 2008.

19. Soreide K, Soreide JA. Bile duct cyst as precursor to biliary tract cancer. *Ann Surg Oncol*, 2007; 14: 1200–1211.

20. Olbourne N A. Choledochal cysts: A review of the cystic anomalies of the biliary tree. *Annals of the Royal College of Surgeons of England*, 1975; 56: 26–32.

21. Savader SJ, Benenati JF, Venbrux AC, Mitchell SE, Widbus DM, Cameron JL, Floyd A. Osterman Jr FA. Choledochal Cysts: Classification and Cholangiographic Appearance. *AJR*, 156: 327–331, February 1991.

22. Kaneyama K, Yamataka A, Urao M, Kobayashi H, Lane GJ, Miyano T. An extremely rare case of symptomatic right hepatic duct diverticulum located outside the liver. *Pediatr Surg Int*, 2005; 21: 1023–1026.

23. Tashiro S, Imaizumi T, Ohkawa H, Okada A, Katoh T, Kawaharada Y, et al. Pancreaticobiliary maljunction: retrospective and nationwide survey in Japan. *J Hepatobiliary Pancreat Surg*, 2003; 10: 345–351.

24. Gorenstein L, Strasberg SM. Etiology of choledochal cysts: two instructive cases. *Can J Surg*, 1985; 28: 363–367.

25. Saing H, Chan KL, Mya GH, Cheng W, Fan ST, Chan FL. Cutaneous stoma in the Roux limb of hepaticojejunostomy (hepaticocutaneous jejunostomy): useful access for intrahepatic stone extraction. *J Pediatr Surg*, 1996; 31: 247–250.

26. Scudamore CH, Hemming AW, Teare JP, Fache JS, Erb SR. Watkinson AF. Surgical management of choledochal cysts. *Am J Surg*, 1994; 167: 497–500.

27. Sarin YK, Sengar M, Puri AS. Forme fruste choledochal cyst. *Indian Pediatr*, 2005; 42: 1153–5.

28. Sarris GE, Tsang D. Choledochocele: case report, literature review and a proposed classification. *Surgery*, 1989; 105: 408–14.

29. Bancroft JD, Bucuvalas JC, Ryckman FC, Dudgeon DL, Saunders RC, Schwarz KB. Antenatal diagnosis of choledochal cyst. *J Pediatr Gastroenterol Nutr*, 1994; 18: 142–5.

30. Lee HC, Yeung CY, Chang PY, Sheu JC, Wang NL. Dilatation of the biliary tree in children: sonographic diagnosis and its clinical significance. *J Ultrasound Med*, 2000; 19: 177–82.

31. Hua MC, Chao HC, Lien R, Lai JY, Lai MW, Man-Shan Kong MS. The Different Clinical and Liver Pathological Characteristics between the Newborns and Infants with Choledochal Cysts. *Chang Gung Med J*, 2009; 32: 198–203.

32. Ueno S, Hirakawa H, Yokoyama S, Imaizumi T, Makuuchi H. Tokai Emergent biliary drainage for choledochal cyst. *J Exp Clin Med*, 2005; 30 (1): 1–6.

33. Irie H, Honda H, Jimi M, Yokohata K, Chijiiwa K, Kuroiwa T, et al. Value of MR cholangiopancreatography in evaluating choledochal cysts. *Am J Roentgenol*, 1998; 171: 1381–5.

34. Saluja SS, Mishra PK, Nayeem M, Nag HH. Choledochal Cyst with Chronic Pancreatitis: Presentation and Management. *J Pancreas*, 2010; 11 (6): 601–603.

35. Prabakaran S, Kumaran N, Regunanthan SR, et al. Spontaneous biliary perforation in a child with features of Ivemark syndrome. *Pediatr Surg Int*, 2000; 16: 109–10.

36. Jan YY, Chen HM, Chen MF. Malignancy in choledochal cysts. *Hepatogastroenterology*, 2000; 47: 337–40.

37. Bloustein PA. Association of carcinoma with congenital cystic conditions of the liver and bile ducts. *Am J Gastroenterol*, 1977; 67: 40–6.

38. Sharma SB, Chandra S, Gupta V. Spontaneous biliary perforation: a rare entity in late infancy and childhood. *Indian Journal of Pediatric*, 2003; 70 (10): 829–831.

39. Gupta V, Sharma SB. Spontaneous perforation of choledochal cyst: A case report and review of literature. *J MGIMS*, Sep 2005; 10 (2): 49–51.

40. Liu CL, Fan ST, Lo CM, Lam CM, Poon RT, Wong J. Choledochal cysts in adults. *Arch Surg*, 2002; 137: 465–8.

41. Yamataka A, Kato Y. *In* Chapter on *Choledochal Cyst*. Puri P and Hollwarth M. **Paediatric Surgery: Diagnosis and Management**. Springer-Verlag Berlin Heidelberg, 2009: 545–55.

42. Mathias JR, Fernandez A, Sninsky CA, Clench MH, Davis RH. Nausea, vomiting, and abdominal pain after Roux-en-Y anastomosis: motility of the jejunal limb. *Gastroenterology*, New York, 1985; 88 (1 Pt 1): 101–107.

43. Martínez MG, Reyes DHE. César Roux: The surgeon and his anastomosis. *Cir Gen*, 2005; 27 (2): 171–5.

Research Paper
(Abstract)

BACKGROUND

Choledochal cyst is an aneurysmal dilatation of the biliary tree involving either extrahepatic or intrahepatic biliary ducts or both, presenting primarily in infants and young children. It is a potentially serious disease with a wide spectrum of presentation. A correct diagnosis and early surgical treatment are important because of the postoperative complications including malignant degeneration. We present our experience with a series of patients with choledochal cyst and discuss its surgical management, with emphasis on reducing the intraoperative and postoperative morbidity.

AIMS

To present the current modality of surgical treatments i.e. complete excision with Roux-en-Y hepaticojejunostomy and Lilly's procedure, and derive appropriate management recommendations in patients of choledochal cyst.

PATIENTS AND METHODS

A prospective study conducted in the department of Paediatric Surgery, SMS Medical College, Jaipur between May 2007 to May 2010 is presented. The study included 55 cases of choledochal cyst. Clinical and surgical details of these patients were recorded. Patients were followed up for 3 to 6 years duration.

RESULTS

The results of the study are summarized in Table 1 to Table 5. There were 55 patients, 30 (54.5%) boys and 25 (45.5%) girls, with male-to-female ratio of 1.2 : 1. The age of patients

Gupta R, Sharma SB, Soni V, Mathur P. Management dilemma with choledochal cyst in paediatric patients: a single institution experience. CIBTech Journal of Surgery, 2014; 3 (1): 27–37.

ranged from newborn to 12 years. Maximum number of patients, 17 (30.9%) were between 5–7 years of age, while 43 (78.2%) patients presented younger than 7 years of age. Jaundice was the most common initial symptom, present in 36 (65.5%) patients. Eight patients (14.5%) had the triad of jaundice, abdominal pain and palpable mass.

PRENATAL DIAGNOSIS

Prenatal diagnosis was not performed in any of the 55 patients. 48 (87.2%) patients were diagnosed by sonography of the abdomen. CT scan of the abdomen was carried out in 54 (98.2%) patients in order to corroborate the diagnosis. Endoscopic retrograde cholangio-pancreatography was carried out in one patient because of recurrent multiple episode of biliary colic, gallstones and dilatation of the biliary tract. It indicated an abnormal common hepatic duct and ERCP stenting was performed. A long pancreaticobiliary common channel was, however, not demonstrated in any of our cases, as the radiologists probably did not look specifically for this anomaly.

OPERATIVE PROCEDURE

Operative procedure was carried out in 52 cases. Age of patients ranged from 5 months to 12 years. 27 (52%) patients with type I underwent excision of the extrahepatic duct, chole-cystectomy and Roux-en-Y hepaticojejunostomy, including one patient with type II (because of the broad base of the cyst), and one patient with type IV cyst. Lilly's procedure was performed in 25 (48%) patients, with cyst being adherent to the portal vein. Concomitant hepatic biopsies were carried out in 4 (7.7%) patients.

POST-OPERATIVE COMPLICATIONS

Post-operative complications were observed in 15 (28.8%) cases. The early post-operative complications (< 3 months postoperatively) were observed in 5 (9.6%) cases. Anastomotic biliary fistula in one case was managed conservatively with reinsertion of sub-hepatic drain. Postoperative intussusception in one patient was managed by peroperative manual reduction. 2 (3.6%) patients presented with cholangitis, managed medically (antibiotics and ursodeoxycholic acid). Burst abdomen seen in one case was treated with tension suturing and it was the only complication seen in patients undergoing Lilly's procedure.

LATE COMPLICATIONS

Late complications (3 months – 3 years postoperatively) were observed in 10 (19.2%) patients. They were biochemical liver dysfunction in 4 patients, managed medically. Recurrent abdominal pain was seen in 2 cases. Residual lithiasis in the hepatic duct present in 1 case was managed with redo-hepaticojejunostomy. Portal hypertension and chronic pancreatitis was present in 1 case each. Internal hernias of the small bowel seen in one female patient 3 years after the procedure and was managed surgically successfully. All the late complications were seen in the patients who underwent total excision, while none in patients with Lilly's procedure. There were no patient deaths during the first 30 days postoperatively, so there was no operative mortality. None of the patients had malignant transformation of the residual cyst wall. Out of the 52 patients who were operated, 30 patients have been lost to follow up but the remainder, 22 patients, are well after 3–6 years.

Distribution of patients as per type of choledochal cyst

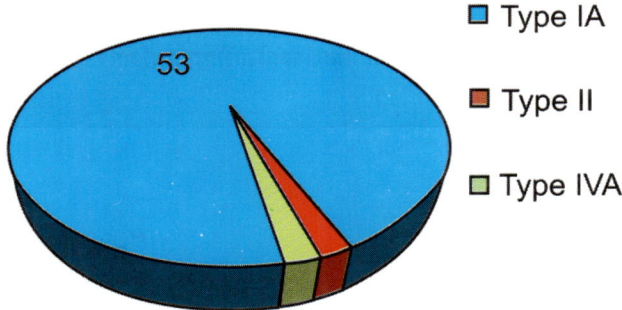

- □ Type IA
- ■ Type II
- □ Type IVA

Table 1. Frequency of type of choledochal cyst according to Todani's classification

Type of cyst	Number of patients (%age)
IA	53 (96.36)
II	01 (1.8)
IVA	01 (1.8)
Total	55 (100)

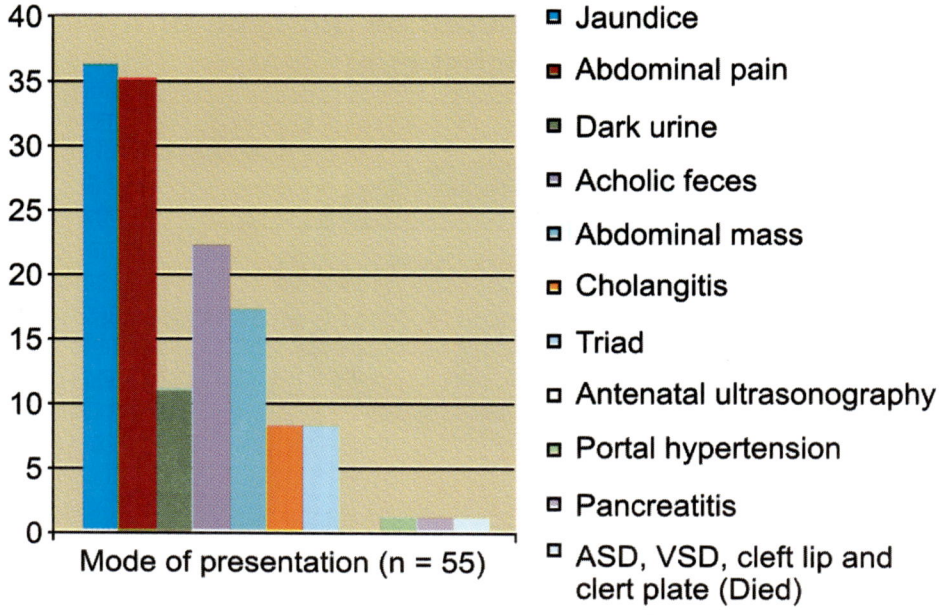

Mode of presentation (n = 55)

- Jaundice
- Abdominal pain
- Dark urine
- Acholic feces
- Abdominal mass
- Cholangitis
- Triad
- Antenatal ultrasonography
- Portal hypertension
- Pancreatitis
- ASD, VSD, cleft lip and clert plate (Died)

Table 2. Presentation of choledochal cyst, out of 55 patients

Mode of presentation	Number (%)
Jaundice	36 (65.5%)
Abdominal pain	35 (63.6%)
Dark urine	11 (20%)
Acholic feces	22 (40%)
Abdominal mass	17 (30.9%)
Cholangitis	08 (14.5%)
Triad	08 (14.5%)
Antenatal ultrasonography	0
Portal hypertension	01 (1.8)
Pancreatitis	01 (1.8)
ASD, VSD, cleft lip and cleft palate (Died)	01 (1.8)

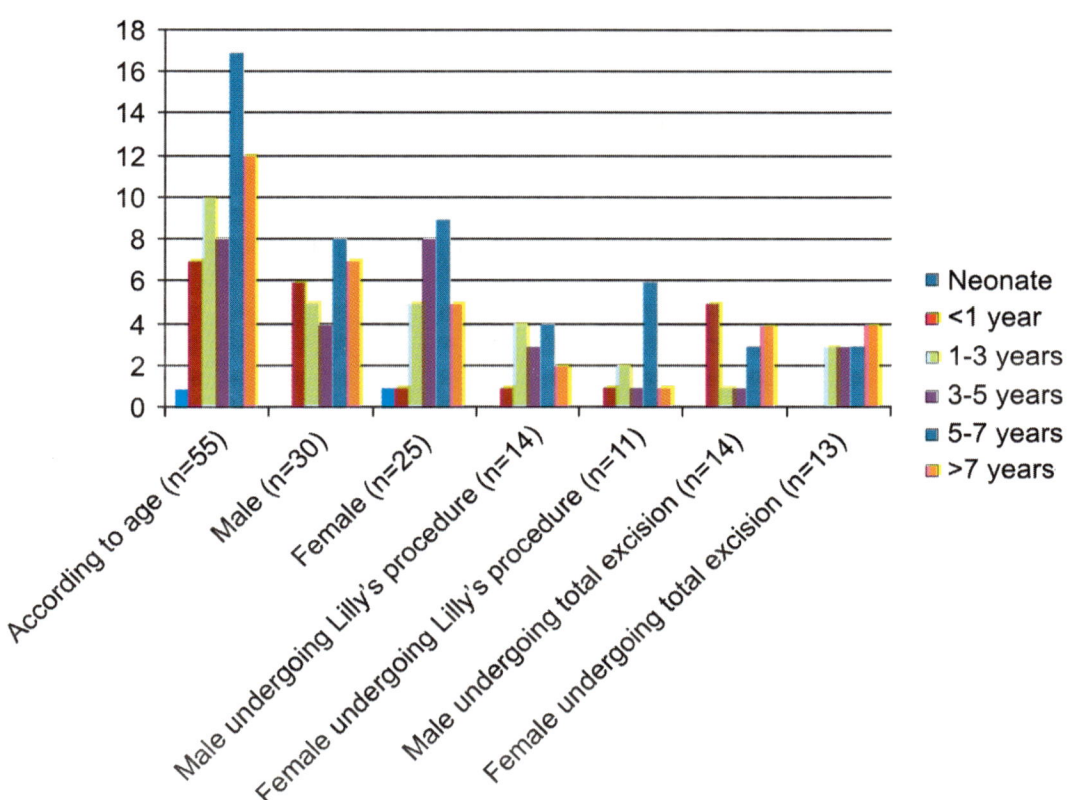

Table 3. Distribution of patients, surgical procedure, according to the age at diagnosis

Age (years)	Number of patients (%age)	Male (Boys)	Female (Girls)	Male Lilly'	Female Lilly's	Male Total excision	Female Total excision
Neonate	1 (1.8)	0	1	0	0	0	0
< 1 year	7 (12.7)	6	1	1	1	5	0
1–3	10 (18.2)	5	5	4	2	1	3
3–5	8 (14.5)	4	4	3	1	1	3
5–7	17 (30.9)	8	9	4	6	3	3
> 7	12 (21.8)	7	5	2	1	4	4
Total	55 (100)	30 (54.5)	25 (45.5)	14	11	14	13
				25 (48%)		27 (52%)	
		55 (100%)		52 (100%)			

Early complications

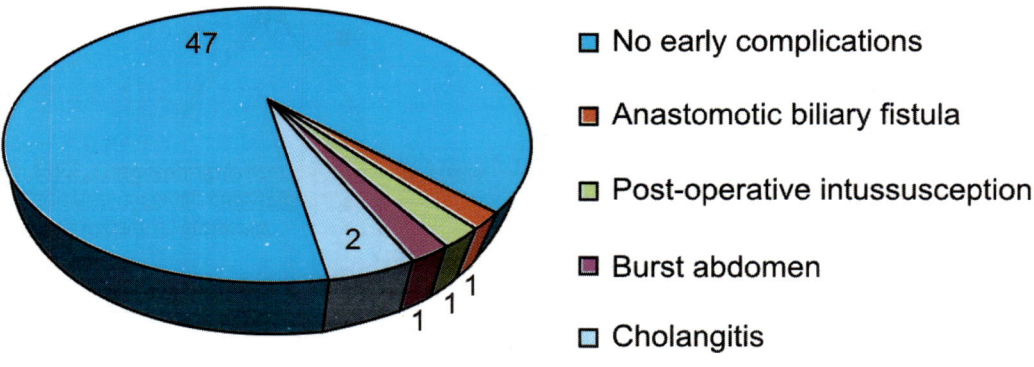

Table 4. Early post-operative complications (< 3 months postoperatively), out of 52 patients

Early complications	N
Anastomotic biliary fistula	1
Post-operative Intussusception	1
Burst abdomen	1
Cholangitis	2
Total	5 (9.6%)

Late complications

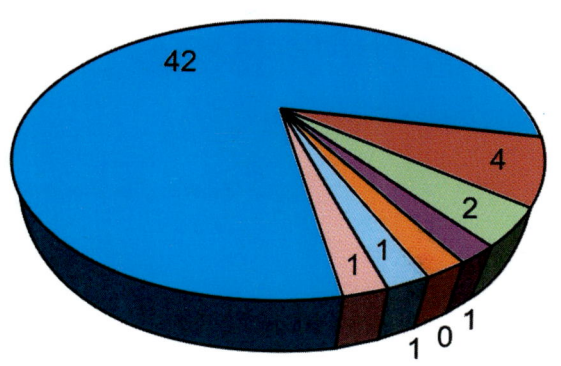

- 🟦 No late complications
- 🟫 Biochemical liver dysfunction
- 🟩 Recurrent abdominal pain
- 🟪 Residual lithiasis in the hepatic duct
- 🟦 Common bile duct adenocarcinoma
- 🟧 Chronic pancreatitis
- ◼️ Portal hypertension
- 🟪 Internal hernias of the small bowel

Table 5. Late complications (3 months – 3 years postoperatively), out of 52 patients

Late complications	N
Biochemical liver dysfunction	4
Recurrent abdominal pain	2
Residual lithiasis in the hepatic duct	1
Common bile duct adenocarcinoma	0
Chronic pancreatitis	1
Portal hypertension	1
Internal hernias of the small bowel	1
Total	10 (19.2%)

Note: We want to humbly accept that wound infection and Seroma were not included in the complications, owing to the fact that, these complications were not recorded in our patients. We again regret for not having included them in the study.

Spontaneous Perforation of Choledochal Cyst
A Case Report and Review of Literature

Vipul Gupta, SB Sharma

ABSTRACT

Spontaneous perforation of choledochal cyst is described in a 9-month-old female infant presented with progressive abdominal distension, low grade fever, acholic stools and jaundice. Abdominal paracentesis suggested presence of bile and precipitated surgery. Surgical exploration revealed sterile biliary peritonitis and a perforated type I choledochal cyst. Primary cyst excision resulted in satisfactory recovery. Authors review their experience with this rare entity and the pertinent literature.

Keywords: Choledochal cyst, Spontaneous perforation, Infants

Introduction

Spontaneous perforation of choledochal cyst being extremely uncommon in paediatric age group warrants recognition of its typical clinical features and management protocol[1,2]. Although an incidence of 1.8% to 2.1% has been reported in handful of reported cases in English literature but its aetiopathogenesis still remains unclear[3,4]. To become proficient in diagnosis of this rare entity an awareness of its clinical presentation characterized by features of subacute peritonitis and biliary obstruction is thus mandatory. Thus, we herein review our experience with a similar case with the aim to make physicians aware of such unusual complication of choledochal cyst so that associated undue high morbidity could be prevented by an early diagnosis and appropriate management.

Case Report

A 9-month-old female infant presented with progressive abdominal distension, a low grade fever, acholic stools and jaundice for the last two days. The patient appeared active and alert

Paper published in *J MGIMS*, Sept. 2005, Vol. 10, No. (ii), 49–51.

with pulse rate of 140/min, dehydration, mild icterus and low grade fever of 100°F. The abdomen was distended and non-tender but liver was palpable 3 cm below the costal margin. DRE suggested acholic stools.

On lab. investigations, the infant had Hb of 10 gm%. Total leucocyte count of 13000/mm^3, serum bilirubin of 2.7 mg/dl, SGOT 175 U/L, SGPT 180 U/L, ALP 250 U/L and a normal renal function tests. Ultrasonography suggested free fluid in peritoneal cavity and hepatomegaly. Abdominal paracentesis revealed sterile bile stained ascitic fluid which precipitated surgery.

After preoperative stabilisation the patient was taken up for laparotomy. Abdominal exploration revealed approximately 500 ml of bile stained ascites with type 1 choledochal cyst and inflammatory changes at porta. A small perforation was present on the anterior wall of choledochal cyst just near junction of bile duct and common hepatic duct. Since dissection at porta appeared feasible, complete excision of choledochal cyst was accomplished by Lilly's technique. The histopathological examination confirmed diagnosis of choledochal cyst. The ascitic fluid was sterile on culture examination. The postoperative period remained uneventful and the patient recovered satisfactorily. Presently, the patient is doing well on follow-up for the last 8 months.

DISCUSSION

Among biliary tract disorders, spontaneous perforation of choledochal cyst is an extremely uncommon in paediatric age group[1]. To the best of our knowledge, among a handful of such reported cases this rare entity has scarcely been discussed in Indian literature till date[1-6]. Moreover, an undue high morbidity associated with its delayed diagnosis and treatment primarily as a result of subtle clinical presentation demands its recognition as a separate clinical entity.

The aetiopathogeneses of spontaneous perforation of choledochal cyst is still unclear mainly owing to its rarity[2-4]. As experienced in the present and a few reported cases the perforation usually occurs in the anterior wall near junction of cystic duct and common hepatic duct[1,2,3,5]. So, the theory of vascular insufficiency due to suboptimal blood supply to this area appears to be the most acceptable aetiological factor resulting in spontaneous perforation of choledochal cyst[1,5,6.] Still few investigators have attributed occurrence of spontaneous perforation of choledochal cyst to reflux of pancreatic juice due to pancreatico-biliary malunion which results in epithelial irritation and subsequently perforation especially in infancy as a result of underlying mural immaturity[2].

As sterile biliary peritonitis is well tolerated by infants, so these patients are usually active, alert and accept feed normally during early course of disease[7]. The clinical presentation in the present case is typical replica of the clinical features being described by most authors in the available literature. The clinical presentation in such infants is insidious and heralded by features of subacute peritonitis and partial biliary obstruction in the form of progressive abdominal distension, low grade fever, mild icterus, and acholic stools[1-3,5].

Laboratory investigations are usually nonspecific and contribute little towards diagnosis. The presence of radiotracer in the peritoneal cavity on cholescintigraphy confirms the diagnosis[1,2]. As experienced in the present case presence of bile on abdominal paracentesis proves to be a useful diagnostic modality in the absence of radiotracer studies.

The treatment of spontaneous perforation of choledochal cyst is primarily surgical. A review of literature suggests that the treatment of spontaneous perforation of choledochal cyst is essentially a staged procedure mainly due to marked extensive portal inflammation, which usually makes extensive surgery both difficult and hazardous. So, a few reported cases have been managed successfully by peritoneal lavage and external biliary drainage followed by cyst excision as a second stage procedure[1-3]. But as experienced in the present case, we feel that the cyst excision with hepaticojejunostomy can be performed successfully in cases where adhesions at porta hepatica are not so extensive so as to make dissection hazardous, Moreover, Lilly's approach as practised in the present case appears to be very useful surgical technique in facilitating the primary excision of the cyst and thus preventing the morbidity associated with staged procedures.

Thus, we conclude that although rare but perforated choledochal cyst should be considered as an important aetiological factor in differential diagnosis of infants presenting with features of biliary peritonitis. Further, we recommend primary corrective surgery in cases where surgical dissection can be performed safely so that morbidity associated with staged procedures could be avoided.

REFERENCES

1. Wagholikar GB, Chetri K, Yochha SK, Sikora SS. Spontaneous perforation – a rare complication of choledochal cyst. *Ind J Gastroenterology*, 2004; 23: 111–112.
2. Ando K, Miyano T, Kohno S, Takamizawa S, Lane G. Spontaneous perforation of choledochal cyst: a study of 13 cases. *Eur J Pediatr Surg*, 1998; 8: 23–5.
3. Ando H, Ito T, Watanabe Y, Seo T, Kaneko K. Nagaya M. Spontaneous perforation of choledochal cyst. *J Am Coll Surg*, 1995; 181 (2): 125–128.
4. Yamaguchi M. Congenital choledochal cyst: Analysis of 1433 patients in the Japanese literature. *Am J Surg*, 1980; 140: 653–657.
5. Stringer MD, Dhawan A, Davenport M, Mieli-Vergani G, Mowat AP, Howard ER. Choledochal cyst: lessons from a 20 year experience. *Arch Dis Child*, 1995; 73 (6): 528–531.
6. Broto J, Bertron JM, Ochoa JB, Enriquez G. Bile peritonitis caused by idiopathic perforation of choledochal cyst. *Arch Fr Pediatr*, 1986; 43 (10): 785–787.
7. Snyder WH, Chaffin L. Cholelithiasis and perforation of the gallbladder in an infant with recovery. *JAMA*, 1952; 149: 1645–1646.

MCQs
Let's check what we have imbibed

1. False about choledochal cyst is:
   - I. Always extrahepatic
   - II. It is common in Japan
   - III. Alanso-Lej et al. classified it into three main types, type I–III
   - IV. Drainage is the treatment of choice

   - (a) II, IV
   - (b) I, IV
   - (c) III, IV
   - (d) I, III

2. True about choledochocele:
   - (a) Type II
   - (b) Type III
   - (c) Type IV
   - (d) Type V

3. Todani classified choledochal cyst on the basis of:
   - (a) U.S.G findings
   - (b) C.T. findings
   - (c) Cholangiography findings
   - (d) Pathology findings

4. Choledochal cyst is explained by:
   - (a) Babbit's theory
   - (b) Todani's theory
   - (c) Boyden's theory
   - (d) Tandler's theory

5. False about choledochal cyst:
   (a) APBDJ (Anomalous Pancreaticobiliary Ductal Junction) is associated with it.
   (b) Embryonic malformation
   (c) Long common channel is associated with it.
   (d) Forme fruste Choledochal cyst is APBDJ with ruptured Choledochal cyst.

6. False about choledochal cyst:
   (a) Type III cyst may be a biliary duplication cyst.
   (b) Type III is also k/a choledochocele
   (c) Type IV-A cysts are more common in children
   (d) Reovirus was detected in patients with choledochal cyst

7. The classical triad of choledochal cyst are except:
   (a) Abdominal pain, Jaundice, Fever
   (b) Right hypochondrial mass, Jaundice, Fever
   (c) Right hypochondrial mass, Abdominal pain, Jaundice
   (d) Abdominal pain, Right hypochondrial mass, Fever

8. Lumps which disappear and reappear are except:
   (a) Choledochal cyst
   (b) Hydronephrosis
   (c) Transient intussusception
   (d) Mesenteric cyst

9. False regarding choledochal cyst is:
   (a) Secondary biliary cirrhosis is common in children > 2 years
   (b) Direct compression of is the mechanism responsible for the development of portal hypertension
   (c) Extrahepatic biliary obstruction is a cause for secondary biliary cirrhosis
   (d) Portal vein thrombosis may lead to cirrhosis.

10. False regarding choledochal cyst is:
    (a) Serum amylase may be raised
    (b) MRCP is investigation of choice
    (c) HIDA scan is noninvasive
    (d) ERCP is screening test

11. Choledochal cyst is a risk factor for all except:
    (a) Biliary tree including liver
    (b) Duodenum
    (c) Jejunum
    (d) Pancreas

12. False regarding choledochal cyst rupture is:
    (a) It is rare
    (b) Site of rupture is often at the junction of cystic duct and CBD.
    (c) Roux-en-Y hepaticojejunostomy is treatment of choice
    (d) External bile drainage is safe

13. False regarding malignancy in choledochal cyst is:
    (a) Posterior wall of the cyst is most frequent site
    (b) Bile stasis is predisposing factor
    (c) Pancreatic juice reflux secondary to APBDJ is predisposing factor
    (d) It is usually resectable

14. False regarding malignancy in choledochal cyst is:
    (a) Adenocarcinoma is most frequent type
    (b) It is commonly seen in children
    (c) It is common with cyst enteric anastomosis
    (d) Chronic mucosal inflammation is predisposing factor

15. Ohkuma's classification is for the assessment of:
    (a) APBDJ
    (b) Choledochal cyst
    (c) Liver fibrosis
    (d) None of the above

16. Differential diagnosis of choledochal cyst are:
    (a) Uncorrectable biliary atresia
    (b) Pancreatic cystic lesions
    (c) Congenital biliary stricture
    (d) Pseudocyst

17. True about Caroli's disease:
    I. Type III
    II. Type V
    III. String of beads appearance
    IV. Associated with APBDJ

    (a) II, IV
    (b) I, IV
    (c) III, IV
    (d) II, III

18. Ultrasound findings of choledochal cyst are except:
    (a) Screening test
    (b) Echogenic mass in the region of the porta hepatis
    (c) It evaluates the entire intrahepatic and extrahepatic biiary system
    (d) Diagnosis of APBDJ is its limitation

19. True about recurrent cholangitis in choledochal cyst are except:
    (a) May lead to portal vein thrombosis
    (b) ERCP is diagnostic
    (c) Lily's procedure is performed
    (d) Cyst is densely adherent to PV.

20. All are true about choledochal cyst except:
    (a) MRCP is investigation of choice
    (b) HIDA is an investigation of choice for neonatal jaundice

(c) HIDA scan may diagnose bile leak from cyst rupture

(d) ERCP is confirmatory and therapeutic for APBDJ and type III cyst.

21. All are true about ERCP in type III cyst except:
    (a) Cobrahead appearance.
    (b) Diagnostic and therapeutic in large cysts
    (c) It is an invasive technique
    (d) Acute pancreatitis is a known complication

22. Ultrasound findings of choledochal cyst are:
    (a) Hyperechoic lesion
    (b) Anechoic lesion
    (c) Ill-defined lesion
    (d) None of the above

23. All are true about choledochal cyst except:
    (a) Well-defined non-enhancing cystic lesion
    (b) Well-defined enhancing cystic lesion
    (c) MRCP images are T2 signal
    (d) Hyperintense lesion on MRCP.

24. All are false about surgery for antenatally diagnosed choledochal cyst except:
    (a) After 1 year
    (b) Fetal surgery
    (c) After 3 months
    (d) Between 1–3 months

25. All are true about choledochal cyst except:
    (a) On exploration may have a variant of extrahepatic biliary atresia
    (b) Early surgery is recommended
    (c) Liver fibrosis progresses much faster in the newborn
    (d) Roux-en-Y hepaticojejunostomy should not be attempted in patients with previous cystenterostomy

26. All are true about aggressive treatment of choledochal cyst except:
    (a) Predisposing factor for malignancy
    (b) Cholecystectomy may or may not be performed
    (c) Intrapancreatic portion of the cyst is excised
    (d) Disconnection is performed between biliary tree and pancreatic duct system.

27. True about distal extent of resection of choledochal cyst except:
    (a) The mucosa of the intrapancreatic portion of the cyst should be stripped
    (b) The distal bile duct stump should be double-suture ligated
    (c) Division of cyst is done proximal to the pancreatic duct
    (d) None of the above.

28. All are true about choledochal cyst except:
    (a) After excision, intrahepatic ducts should be lavaged with saline
    (b) Endoscopic treatment is the method of choice for uncomplicated type III cyst.

(c) Surgical excision is treatment of choice for type III cyst.

(d) In type IVA cyst intrahepatic dilatations are always left-sided.

29. All are true about choledochal cyst except:
    (a) Roux-en-Y hepaticojejunostomy is treatment of choice for type V cyst.
    (b) Hepatic lobectomy for disease limited to one hepatic lobe
    (c) Liver transplantation for bilobar disease
    (d) After perforation of choledochal cyst initial external biliary drainage is safe

30. All are true about recurrent bouts of cholangitis, and pancreatitis in choledochal cyst except:
    (a) In these patients portal vein injury is a known complication
    (b) In Lilly's procedure mucosectomy is performed
    (c) Laparoscopic technique of cyst excision is a relative contraindication
    (d) Lilly's procedure can be performed with laparoscopic technique

31. Regarding postoperative stricture in choledochal cyst, all are true except:
    (a) Hepaticojejunostomy is better
    (b) Choledochojejunostomy is preferred
    (c) Cholangitis is predisposing factor
    (d) Postoperative biliary leak is a predisposing factor

32. Regarding risk of malignancy in choledochal cyst, all are true except:
    (a) Increases with age
    (b) Malignancy is never seen with type III cyst
    (c) In forme fruste type, malignancy is seen in the gallbladder
    (d) It may be seen after Roux-en-Y hepaticojejunostomy

33. All are true about ERCP in choledochal cyst except:
    (a) Invasive investigation
    (b) APBDJ is evaluated
    (c) Important investigation postoperatively after Roux-en-Y hepaticojejunostomy
    (d) Acute pancreatitis is a known complication with ERCP.

ANSWERS WITH REFERENCES (TOPICS)

1. b, Incidence and treatment
2. b, Todani modification of Alonso-Lej classification system
3. c, Todani modification of Alonso-Lej classification system
4. a, Embryology of pancreaticobiiary ductal system and aetiology
5. d, Aetiology
6. c, Aetiology and clinical presentation
7. c, Clinical presentation
8. d, Clinical presentation
9. a, Complications
10. d, Investigations
11. c, Complications

12. c, Complications
13. d, Complications
14. b, Complications
15. c, Pathology
16. a, Differential diagnosis
17. d, Investigations
18. b, Investigations
19. b, Investigations and Lilly's procedure
20. d, Investigations and procedure of choledochal cyst excision
21. b, Investigations and procedure of choledochal cyst excision
22. b, Investigations
23. b, Investigations and procedure of choledochal cyst excision
24. d, Surgical management
25. d, Surgical management
26. b, Operative procedures
27. d, Surgical management
28. c, Surgical management
29. a, Surgical management
30. c, Lilly's procedure
31. b, Postoperative complications
32. b, Malignant change after cyst excision
33. c, Postoperative follow-up

Paediatric Drug Dosage

Drug	Dose	Maximum dose	Formulation
	ANTIBIOTICS		
	Aminoglycosides		
Amikacin	15–20 mg/kg/d BD	1.5 gm/d	Inj 100, 250, 500/2 ml
Streptomycin	20–40 mg/kg/d BD	0.75–1 g/d	Inj 0.75, 1 gm vial
Gentamycin	5–7.5 mg/kg/d	—	10 & 40 mg/ml amp
Netilimycin	5–7.5 mg/kg/d	—	10, 25, 50, 100 mg/ml
	Cephalosporins (Oral)		
Cefaclor	20–40 mg/kg/d TDS	2 g/d	125, 250, 500 mg tab; 125 & 187 mg/5 ml syp
Cefadroxil	30 mg/kg/d BD	2 g/d	Tab 500, 1 gm; Syp odoxil 125/5 ml
Cefprozil	15–30 mg/kg/d BD	1 gm/d	Refzil-o tab 250, 500; Syp 125, 250/5 ml
Cefuroxime	20–30 mg/kg/d BD	1 gm/d	Ceftum 250, 500 mg; Syp 125/5 ml
Cephalexin	25–100 mg/kg/d TDS	4 g/d	Cephaxin 250, 500; Syp 125/5 ml

(Contd.)

Inputs from Dr. Priyanka Golash

Drug	Dose	Maximum dose	Formulation
Cefixime	8 mg/kg/d BD	800 mg/d	Tab 50, 100, 200 DT; Syp 50, 100/5 ml
Cefpodoxime	10 mg/kg/d BD	400 mg/d	Tab 50, 100, 200; Syp 100/5 ml
Cephalosporins (IV)			
Cefazolin	50–100 mg/kg/d QID	500–1 g/d	250, 500, 1 g vial
Cefepime	100 mg/kg/d BD 60 mg/kg/d BD (< 2 mths)	2 g/d	250, 500, 1 g vial
Cefoperazone	100–150 mg/kg/d BD	4 g/d	250, 500, 1, 2 g vial
Cefotaxim	100–150 mg/kg/d TDS	4 g/d	250, 500, 1 g vial
Ceftazidime	100–150 mg/kg/d TDS	6 g/d	250, 500, 1 g vial
Ceftizoxime	100–200 mg/kg/d TDS	6 g/d	250, 1 g vial
Cefuroxime	50–100 mg/kg/d TDS	4.5 g/d	250, 750, 1500 vial
Ceftriaxone	50–75 mg/kg/d BD 100 mg/kg/d (meningitis)	2–4 g/d	125, 250, 500, 1 gm vial
Fluoroquinolines			
Ciprofloxacin	Oral: 20–30 mg/kg/d IV: 10–20 mg/kg/d BD	800 mg/d	Tab 100, 250, 500, 750; Syp 125, 250/5 ml; Inj 100, 200 mg (2 mg/ml)
Levofloxacin	Oral/IV: 10 mg/kg/d OD	500 mg/d	Tab 250, 500; Inj 5 mg/ml
Nalidixic acid	50 mg/kg/d TDS	4 g/d	Tab 500; syp 300/5 ml
Norfloxacin	Oral: 10–15 mg/kg/d BD	400 mg/d	Tab 100, 200, 400, 800; Syp 100 mg/5 ml
Ofloxacin	Oral: 15 mg/kg/d BD IV: 5–10 mg/kg/d BD	800 mg/d	Tab 100, 200, 400; Syp 50, 100 mg/5 ml; Inj 200, 400/100 ml
Pefloxacin	Oral: 12 mg/kg/d BD	800 mg/d	Tab 200, 400
Sparfloxacin	Oral: 4 mg/kg OD	800 mg/d	Tab 100, 200
Lincosamides			
Clindamycin	Oral/IV: 20–30 mg/kg/d TDS	—	Cap 150, 300 mg; Inj 150 mg/ml in 2, 4 ml amp

(Contd.)

Drug	Dose	Maximum dose	Formulation
Lincomycin	Oral: 30–60 mg/kg/d TDS IV: 10–20 mg/kg/d TDS	2 g/d	Cap 250, 500; Syp 125/ml; Inj 300/ml in 1, 2 ml amp

Macrolides			
Azithromycin	10 mg/kg/d OD; Enteric fever: 20 mg/kg/d for 7–14 days	500 mg/d	Tab 100, 250, 500; Syp 100, 200/5 ml
Clarithromycin	15 mg/kg/d BD	1 g/d	Tab 250, 500; Syp 125/5 ml
Erythromycin	30–50 mg/kg/d QID	1 g/d	Tab 100, 125, 250, 500; Syp 100, 125 mg/5 ml
Roxithromycin	5–8 mg/kg/d BD	300 mg/d	Tab 50, 150 mg; Syp 50 mg/5 ml

Penicillins			
Amoxicillin	25–50 mg/kg/d TDS	2 g/d	Cap 250, 500; DT 125, 250; Syp 125/5 ml; Drops 100/ml
Amoxicillin + Clavulanate	Oral: 30 mg/kg/d TDS IV: 90 mg/kg/d TDS	Oral: 1.5 g/d IV: 4.8 gm/d	Tab 375 (250 + 125), 625 (500 + 125), 1000 (875 + 125); Syp 125, 200, 400/5 ml; Drops 80/ml; Inj 150, 300, 600, 1.2 g
Ampicillin	Oral/IV: 100–200 mg/kg/d QID	2 g/d	Cap 250, 500; DT 125, 250; Syp 125/5 ml; Drops 100/ml; Inj 250, 500 vial
Ampicillin + Sulbactam	IV: 100–200 mg/kg/d	—	Inj 1.5 g (1 + 0.5); Tab 375
Cloxacillin	Oral/IV: 50–100 mg/kg/d QID	2 g/d	Cap 250, 500; Syp 125/5 ml (with ampicillin); Cap 250 + 250; Syp 125 + 125/5 ml; Inj 250, 500 vial
Piperacillin + Tazobactum	IV: 300 mg/kg/d TDS	12 g/d	1.125, 2.25, 4.5 g
Ticarcillin + Clavulunate	IV: 240–320 mg/kg/d TDS	12 g/d	Inj 3.1 (3 g + 100 mg)

(Contd.)

Drug	Dose	Maximum dose	Formulation
Penicillin G (Aqueous)	1–2 lac IU/kg/dose QID	120 lac IU/d	Inj benzyl penicillin 5, 10 lac IU/vial
Penicillin G (Benzathine)	12 lac IU (every 21 days) > 6 years; 6 lac (< 6 years)	—	Inj 6, 12, 24 lac IU

Carbapenams			
Imipenem/Cilastatin	60–100 mg/kg/d QID	2 g/d	Inj 250 + 250; 500 + 500
Meropenam	60 mg/kg/d TDS Neonatal sepsis: 20 mg/kg/dose BD Neonatal meningitis: 40 mg/kg/dose TDS	3 g/d	Inj 500, 1000 mg

Miscellaneous			
Co-trimoxazole	Oral/IV: 5–8 mg/kg/d TMP; 25–50 mg/kg/d SMX; 20 mg/kg/d TMP for *P. jiroveci*; single dose 1–3 mg/kg/d TMP for UTI prophylaxis	—	Tab 80 + 400; 160 + 800 (DS) 20 + 100 (pediatric); Syp 40 + 200/5 ml
Aztreonam	90–300 mg/kg/d TDS IV/IM	8 gm/d	Inj 250, 500, 1, 2 gm vial
Colistin	5–15 mg/kg/d TDS	300 mg/d	Syp 12.5, 25 mg/5 ml
Doxycycline	5 mg/kg/d BD	200 mg/d	Tab 100, 200; Syp 25, 50 mg/ml
Linezolid	30 mg/kg/d TDS (oral/IV)	1.2 g/d	Inj 200, 600 (in 100, 300 ml vials) [2 mg/ml]; Tab 600 mg; Syp 100/5 ml
Teicoplanin	10 mg/kg q 12 hr for 3 doses then OD IM/IV	800 mg/d	Inj 200, 400 mg vials
Vancomycin	45 mg/kg/d TDS; 60 mg/kg/d TDS (CNS infections)	2 g/d	500,1 gm vial
Nitrofurantoin	5–7 mg/kg/d BD	400 mg/d	Tab 50, 100 mg; Syp 25/5 ml

ANTIMALARIALS			
Artemether	3.2 mg/kg IM (Day 1) then 1.6 mg/kg for next 4 days	80–160 mg/d	Inj 80 mg/ml
Artemether + Lumefantrine (20 + 120 mg)	5–14 kg: 1 tab BD 15–24: 2 tab BD; 25–34: 3 tab BD; > 35: 4 tab BD	—	Tab lumerax 40, 60, 80; Syp 20 + 120/5 ml

(Contd.)

Drug	Dose	Maximum dose	Formulation
Arteether	3.2 mg/kg IM (Day 1) then 1.6 mg/kg for next 4 days	—	Inj 150 mg/2 ml
Artesunate (IV)	IV: 2.4 mg/kg BD (Day 1) then OD for 7 days	—	Inj 60 mg vial
Artesunate (Oral) Pyrimathamine + Sulfadoxine	4 mg/kg/d 1 mg/kg (P) + 20 mg/kg (S)	—	Larinate kit: 50, 100, 200 (Artesunate) + Pyrimethamine 25 + sulfadoxine 500 (single dose on D 1)
Chloroquine	10 mg/kg stat f/b 5 mg/kg at 6, 24, 48 hr; or 10 mg/kg 0, 24 hr; then 5 mg/kg at 48 hr	600 mg f/by 300 mg at 6, 24, 48 hr	Tab 250 (with 150 mg base); Syp 50 mg/5 ml
Primaquine	0.25 mg/kg/d for 14 days (*Pv*); 0.75 mg/kg stat (*Pf*) (Radical cure)	15 mg/d	Tab 2.5, 7.5, 15 mg
Quinine (IV)	20 mg/kg over 4 hrs (loading) in 5% dextrose @ 1 mg/ml f/b 10 mg/kg TDS as 4 hr infusion	—	Inj 300 mg/ml as 2 ml amp
Quinine (Oral)	30 mg/kg/d TDS	2 g/d	Tab 100, 300, 600

Analgesics, Antipyretics & Anti-inflammatory			
Aspirin (Acetyl salicylic acid)	Pain: 30–65 mg/kg/d QID Rheumatic fever: 90–120 mg/kg/d QID; Rheumatoid arthritis: 65–130 mg/kg/d	—	Tab 75 100, 150, 300, 325, 650
Diclofenac	1–3 mg/kg/d (Oral/IV)	150 mg/d	Tab 25, 50, 75, 100, DT 46.5; Inj 75/3 ml
Fentanyl	0.5–5 mcg/kg/dose 1–4 hrly; 1–5 mcg/kg/hr continuous infusion	—	Inj 50 mcg/ml
Ibuprufen	Pain/fever:10–15 mg/kg/dose 4–6 hrly (max 40–60 mg/kg/d JIA: 30–70 mg/kg/d Ductus closure: 10 mg/kg stat f/b 5 mg/kg OD for 2 doses (oral/IV)	1.8 gm/d	Tab 200, 400, 600, 400 + 325 (pcm); Syp 100 + 125 (pcm) [flexon]; Syp 100 + 162.5 (pcm) [Ibugesic plus]
Indomethacin	3 mg/kg/d TDS (oral); Ductus closure: 0.2 mg/kg/dose q 8 hrly for 3 doses	150 mg/d	Cap 25, 50, 75; Inj 1 mg vial
Mefenamic acid	Arthritis: 25 mg/kg/d TDS Fever: 5–8 mg/kg/dose	1.5 g/d	Tab 100 (meftal-P), 250, 500; Syp 100/5 ml; 100 + 250 [pcm]/5 ml (meftagesic DS)

(Contd.)

Drug	Dose	Maximum dose	Formulation
Morphine	0.1–0.2 mg/kg/dose SC (max 15 mg); 2–5 mg/dose for preoperative preparation, post-op pain *Continuous infusion:* Newborn 0.01–0.02 mg/kg/hr; Infants and children: 0.02–0.2 mg/kg/hr	—	Inj 10, 20, 25 mg/ml
Naproxen	JRA: 10–20 mg/kg/d BD Analgesia: 5–7 mg/kg/dose TDS	750 mg/d	Tab 250, 375, 500
Nimesulide	5 mg/kg/d BD	200 mg/d	Tab 50, 100 mg; Syp 50/5 ml
Paracetamol	15 mg/kg/dose 4–6 hrly (Oral/rectal); 5 mg/kg/dose IM	4 gm/d	Tab 500, 650; Syp 125, 250/5 ml; Drops 100/ml (crocin), 150/ml (calpol); Inj 150/ml; Suppository 80, 170
Pentazocine	0.5–1 mg/kg/d QID (oral, IM, IV)	—	Tab 25 mg; 15 + 500 (pcm); Inj 30/ml
Tramadol	50–100 mg q TDS (Avoid < 14 years)	400 mg/d	Tab 50, 100; Inj 50/ml in 1, 2 ml vials

ANTICONVULSANTS			
ACTH	30–40 IU/d IM/SC for 4 wks f/b gradual tapering over 2 wks	—	Inj 40, 50, 60 in/ml
Carbamazepine	10–30 mg/kg/d BD [start with 30–50% of dose]	1000 mg/d	Tab 100, 200, 400; SR 200, 400; Syp 100/5 ml
Clobazam	0.3–1 mg/kg/d BD	60 mg/d	Tab 5, 10, 20 mg
Clonazepam	0.01–0.03 mg/kg/d, increase by 0.25–0.5 mg every 3 days to max 0.2 mg/kg/d	—	Tab 0.5, 2 mg
Diazepam	Status epilepticus: 0.2–0.5 mg/kg/dose (IV/IM/Rectal) Neonatal tetanus: 0.5–5 mg/kg q 2–4 hrly (max 60 mg/kg/d)	—	Inj 10 mg/2 ml [5 mg/ml]
Ethosuximide	15 mg/kg/d increased weekly till 20–40 mg/kg/d BD	< 6 yrs: 500 mg/d > 6 yrs: 1500 mg/d	Tab 250 mg; Syp 250/5 ml
Fosphenytoin (1.5 mg of fosphenytoin is equivalent to 1 mg of phenytoin)	15–20 mg/kg (L) f/b 5 mg/kg (M)	Infusion rate 3 mg/kg/min	Inj 50 mg/ml

(Contd.)

Drug	Dose	Maximum dose	Formulation
Gabapentin (Avoid < 12 yrs)	15 mg/kg/d increased to 30–60 mg/kg/d TDS	—	Cap 300, 400 mg
Lamotrigine	Without valproate: 5–10 mg/kg/d BD; With valproate: 0.5–5 mg/kg/d OD	—	—
Levetiracetam	10 mg/kg/d – increase by 10 mg/kg/week to 60 mg/kg/d	1–3 gm/d	Tab 250, 500, 750, 1000 mg; Syp 100 mg/ml
Lorazepam	0.05–0.1 mg/kg/dose (max 4 mg) rpt once after 10–15 min	—	Inj 2 mg/ml; Inj 10 mg/ml
Midazolam	*Status epilepticus:* 0.2 mg/kg IV bolus f/b 0.1–0.2 mg/kg/hr *Sedation for MV (NB):* 0.2–1 mcg/kg/min (Infants & children): 0.5–3 mcg/kg/min *Sedation:* 0.05–0.1 mg/kg over 2 min may rpt same dose every 2–3 min (total 0.2 mg/kg) *Intranasal:* 0.2 mg/kg	—	Inj 1 mg/ml; 5 mg/ml; Nasal spray: 0.5 mg/ metered dose
Phenobarbitone	(L) 15–20 mg/kg over 15–20 min @ 1 mg/kg/min – additional 5 mg/kg every 15–30 min to a max 30 mg/kg (M) 3–5 mg/kg BD	—	Inj 200 mg/ml – stock solution (dilution in 10 ml NS 20 mg/ml); Syp 20 mg/5 ml; Tab 30, 60 mg, 100 mg
Phenytoin	(L) 15–20 mg/kg @ 1 mg/kg/min (M) 5–8 mg/kg/min BD	—	Inj 50 mg/ml; Tab 50, 100 mg; Syp 30 mg/5 ml
Prednisolone	2 mg/kg/d BD* 2–6 wks – taper over 4–12 wks (Infantile spasms)	—	Tab 5, 10, 20; Syp 5 mg/5 ml, 10 mg/ml
Pyridoxine	50–100 mg/dose IM or rapid IV; 50–100 mg/d (maintenance)	—	Tab 40, 100 mg; Inj 100 mg/ml
Valproate	Initial 10–15 mg/kg then increase by 5–10 mg/kg every week till 60 mg/kg/d SE: 20 mg/kg (L) f/b 5–10 mg/kg/dose TDS (M) @ 20 mg/min	1–2 g/d	Tab 200, 300, 500; Syp 200 mg/5 ml; Inj 100 mg/ml
ANTIHISTAMINICS			
Cetrizine	6 mths – 2 yrs 2.5 mg OD; 2–6 yrs 5 mg OD; > 6 yrs 5–10 mg OD	10–20 mg/d	Tab 5, 10 mg; Syp 5 mg/5 ml

(Contd.)

Drug	Dose	Maximum dose	Formulation
Chlorpheniramine	0.35 mg/kg/d q 4–6 hr 1–6 yrs 1 mg q 4–6 hr 6–12 yrs 2 mg q 4–6 hr > 12 yrs 4 mg q 4–6 hr	4 mg 4–6 hr	Tab 2, 4, 6 mg; Syp 1, 2 mg/5 ml
Cyproheptadine	0.25–0.5 mg/kg/d BD/TDS	2–6 yrs 12 mg/d 7–14 yrs 16 mg/d	Tab 2, 4 mg; Syp 2 mg/5 ml
Hydroxyzine	2 mg/kg/d QID	—	Tab 10, 25 mg; Syp 10 mg/5 ml; Drops 6 mg/ml
Levocetrizine	2–6 yrs 0.125 mg/kg/d OD > 6 yrs 2.5 mg OD	—	Tab 5 mg; Syp 2.5 mg/5 ml
Loratidine	2 yrs 30 kg 5 mg/d > 12 yrs 10 mg/d	—	Tab 10 mg; Syp 5 mg/5 ml
Pheniramine (avil)	0.5 mg/kg/d TDS oral/IV/IM	—	Inj 22.75 mg/ml; Tab 25, 50 mg
Promethazine (Phenargan)	0.25–1 mg/kg/dose 4–6 hrly IM/IV/oral	—	Inj 25 mg/ml; Tab 10, 25 mg; Syp 5 mg/5 ml

ANTIHELMINTHICS & ANTIPROTOZOAL			
Albendazole	*Pinworms, roundworms, hookworm:* 200 mg stat (1–2 yrs); 400 mg stat (> 2 yrs) For roundworms repeat dose after 2 wks; *Strongyloidoses, teniasis, H. nana:* Same dose for 3 days *Giardiasis:* Same dose for 5 days *Hydratid disease:* Same dose twice a day for 28 days; For eradication of hydratid cysts therapy may be repeated after 14 days for total of 3 cycles. *NCC:* 15 mg/kg/d BD for 28 days (on day 3 of starting steroids, which are to be given for total 5 days)	—	Tab 200, 400 mg; Syp 200 mg/5 ml
Nitazoxanide	1–4 yrs – 100 mg BD for 3 days 4–12 yrs – 200 mg BD for 3 days (Giardiasis, E. histolytica, Cryptosporodiosis)	—	Tab 200 DT, 500; Syp 100 mg/5 ml
Metronidazole	Giardiasis: 15–20 mg/kg/d TDS (oral) Amoebiasis: 35–50 mg/kg/d TDS (oral) Anaerobic infections: 20 mg/kg/d TDS (oral/IV)	—	Tab 200, 400 mg; Syp 200 mg/5 ml; Inj 500/100 ml

(Contd.)

Drug	Dose	Maximum dose	Formulation
Ornidazole	40 mg/kg OD for 3 days (giardiasis, amoebiasis)	—	Tab 500 mg
Tinidazole	50–60 mg/kg single dose for 3 days (amoebiasis, giardiasis)	—	Tab 150, 300, 500 mg; Syp 300 mg/5 ml

ANTIHYPERTENSIVES			
Clonidine	15–25 mcg/kg/d TDS/QID	—	Tab 100, 150 mcg
Enalapril	0.1–0.6 mg/kg/d BD/OD	—	Tab 2.5, 5, 10, 20 mg
Labetalol	5–10 mg/kg/d BD (oral); Hypertensive crises: 0.25–1 mg/kg IV over 2 min; Continuous infusion 0.4–3 mg/kg/hr	—	Tab/cap 50, 100, 200 mg; Inj 5 mg/ml, 20 mg/ml
Nifedipine	0.25–0.5 mg/kg/dose 4–6 hrly	10 mg	Cap 5, 10, 20 mg; Tab 10 mg
Propranolol	Hypertension: 0.5–1 mg/kg/d BD Cyanotic spell: 0.5–4 mg/kg/d TDS	—	Tab 10, 40, 80 mg; Inj 1 mg/ml
Sodium nitroprusside	0.5–0.8 mcg/kg/min (50 mg amp dissolved in 1000 ml D 5% to make 50 mcg/ml)	—	Inj 50 mg

ANTIEMETICS & ANTISPASMODICS			
Domperidone	0.2–0.4 mg/kg/dose TDS	—	Tab 5, 10 mg; Syp 5 mg/5 ml; Drops 10 mg/ml
Metoclopramide	0.1 mg/kg/dose TDS (Oral/IM/IV)	—	Tab 10 mg; Syp 5 mg/5 ml; Inj 5 mg/ml
Ondansetron	Oral: < 4 yrs 2 mg q 4 hr 4–11 yrs: 4 mg q 4 hr > 12 yrs: 8 mg q 4 hr IV: 0.15–0.45 mg/kg/dose	—	Syp 2 mg/5 ml; Tab 4, 8 mg; Inj 2 mg/ml
Prochlorperazine (stematil)	0.4 mg/kg/d QID (Oral) IM: Half of oral	—	Tab 5, 25 mg; Inj 12.5 mg/ml
Dicyclomine	6 mths – 2 yrs: 10–20 drops before feeds > 2 yrs: 1 ml q 6 hrly	—	—
Hyosine (Buscopan)	6–12 yrs Oral: 10 mg TDS IM/IV: 10–20 mg bolus	—	Tab 10 mg; Inj 20 mg/ml
Drotaverine	Oral/IV 1–6 yrs: 20 mg TDS > 6 yrs: 40 mg TDS	—	Tab 20, 40 mg; Inj 20 mg/ml

(Contd.)

Drug	Dose	Maximum dose	Formulation
ANTIVIRAL & ANTIFUNGALS			
Acyclovir	HSV encephalitis: IV 10 mg/kg/dose TDS for 14 d Chicken-pox (uncomplicated): [non-pregnant > 13 yrs; Immuno-compromised children > 1 yr] oral 20 mg/kg/dose QID for 5 d Complicated chickenpox: IV 500 mg/sq. m/dose or 10 mg/kg/dose TDS for 7–10 d Herpes zoster (uncomplicated): (oral) 20 mg/kg/dose QID for 5 d Herpes zoster (complicated esp in immunocompromised): (IV) 500 mg/sq. m/dose TDS or 10 mg/kg/dose TDS	800 mg QID	Tab 200, 400, 600 mg; Syp 400 mg/5 ml; Inj 250 mg, 500, 1 gm; Ointment 0.5%
Ganciclovir	Acquired CMV retinitis, pneumonitis, GI infections: 10 mg/kg/d BD for 14–21 d (Induction IV) f/b 5 mg/kg OD (maintainence oral) Prophylaxis of CMV in high risk cases: 10 mg/kg/d BD for 7 days f/b 5 mg/kg/d OD (oral) for 100 d Severe CMV pneumonitis: 10 mg/kg/dose TDS for 14 d	—	Cap 250 mg; Inj 500 mg
Valaganciclovir	CMV prophylaxis (post-trans-plant): 16 mg/kg/dose QID for100 d	—	Tab 250 mg
Oseltamivir	Treatment: < 3 mths: 12 mg BD 3–5 mths: 20 mg BD 6–11mths: 25 mg BD < 15 kg: 30 mg BD 15–23: 45 mg BD 23–40: 60 mg BD > 40: 75 mg BD; Prophylaxis: Same dose OD for 7–10 days	—	Cap 30, 45, 75 mg; Syp 12 mg/ml
Amphotericin-b	(Deoxycholate): 1 mg/kg/d (Liposomal): 5 mg/kg/d [in dextrose 5% over 4–6 hrs]	—	Inj 10, 25, 50 mg
Fluconazole	3–6 mg/kg OD (oral/IV)	12 mg/kg/d	Tab 50, 150, 200 mg Inj 2 mg/ml
Terbinafine	5–8 mg/kg/d OD Upto 20 kg: 62.5 mg OD 20–40 kg: 125 mg OD > 40 kg: 250 mg OD	—	Tab 250 mg

(Contd.)

Drug	Dose	Maximum dose	Formulation
Griseofulvin	10 mg/kg/d BD 20 mg/kg/d BD (for nail lesions) for 6–12 wks	—	Tab 125, 250 mg
Voriconazole	7 mg/kg/d BD (> 1 yr)	—	Tab 50, 200 mg
Caspofungin	50 mg/sq. m/d	—	—

CARDIOTONIC, DIURETIC & ANTICOAGULANT

Adrenaline	*Cardiac arrest (endotracheal/IV):* 0.1 ml/kg/dose (1 : 10000) *Anaphylaxis and bronchial asthma:* 0.01 ml/kg (1 : 1000) IM/SC *Shock:* 0.1–1 mcg/kg/min	—	Inj 1 mg/ml of 1 : 1000 sol
Norepinephrine	0.05–0.1 mcg/kg/min	2 mcg/kg/min	1 mg/ml
Dopamine	5 mcg/kg/min	30 mcg/kg/min	Inj 40 mg/ml
Dobutamine	5–20 mcg/kg/min	—	Inj 25, 50 mg/ml
Digoxin	—	—	—
Vasopressin	0.3–2 mu/kg/min Catecholamine resistant shock/bleeding varices	—	Inj 20 u/ml 10–20 u dissolved in 100–200 ml 5% dextrose
Furesemide	2–8 mg/kg/d BD (oral) 1–4 mg/kg/d BD (IV) 0.1–1 mg/kg/hr (IV infusion)	2–4 mg/kg/dose TDS/QID (oral)	Tab 40 mg, 500 mg; Inj 10 mg/ml
Spironolactone	2–3 mg/kg/d OD	—	Tab 25, 50, 100 mg; Lasilactone cap Frusemide (20 mg) Spironolactone (50 mg)
Acetazolamide	Diuretic: 5 mg/kg/d TDS Hydrocephalus: 20 mg/kg/dose TDS	500 mg/d	Tab 250 mg
Heparin	50 u/kg (bolus) f/b 10–25 u/kg/hr (IV infusion) SC: 25–50 u/kg/dose BD DVT prophylaxis: 5000 u/dose SC BD/TDS until ambulatory (INR 1.5–2.5)	—	Inj 1000, 5000 u/ml 0.83 mg = 100 u
Warfarin	0.05–0.34 mg/kg/d oral/IV	—	Tab 1, 2, 5 mg; Inj 50 mg vial

(Contd.)

Drug	Dose	Maximum dose	Formulation
	**BRONCHODIALATORS**			
Adrenalin	Bronchodialator: 0.01 ml/kg/dose of 1 : 1000 sol (max 0.5 ml) IM Cardiac arrest (IV/Endotracheal): 0.1 ml/kg/dose of 1 : 10000 sol Laryngeal edema (Anaphylaxis): 0.01 ml/kg of 1 : 10000 sol by nebuliser	—	1 mg/ml of 1 : 1000 sol
Aminophylline	15–20 mg/kg/d TDS (oral) Status asthmaticus: 5–7 mg/kg (Loading) f/b 0.5–0.9 mg/kg/hr (Maintainence) Apnea in preterm: 5 mg/kg (L) f/b 2 mg/kg TDS (M)	—	Tab 100 mg; Inj 25 mg/ml
Beclomethasone	Mild persistent asthma: 200–400 mcg/d BD Moderate persistent asthma: 400–800 mcg/d BD Severe persistent asthma: 800–1000 mcg/d BD	—	MDI, rotacap 50, 100, 200 mcg/puff Or cap
Budesonide	Mild persistent asthma: 100–400 mcg/d BD Moderate persistent asthma: 400–600 mcg/d BD Severe persistent asthma: 600–800 mcg/d BD	—	MDI 100, 200 mcg/ puff; Rotacap 100, 200, 400/cap; Respule 0.5, 1 mg in 2 ml
Doxophylline	6 mg/kg/dose BD (only in > 6 yrs)	—	Tab 400 mg; Syp 100 mg/5 ml
Formeterol	12 mcg/dose BD	—	MDI 12 mcg/puff; Rotacap 12 mcg 6 mcg in combination with budesonide
Fluticasone	*Mild persistent asthma:* 50–100 mcg/d; *Moderate persistent asthma:* 100–200 mcg/d; *Severe persistent asthma:* 200–500 mcg/d	—	MDI 25, 50, 125/puff; Rotacap 100, 250, 500/ cap
Salbutamol	0.1 mg/kg/dose TDS (oral) *Asthma exacerbation:* Upto 3 treatments of 2–4 puffs every 20 min f/f 2 puffs q 4–6 hr *Nebulisation:* 0.15 mg/kg/dose q 20 min for 3 times f/b q 4–6 hrly	—	Tab 2, 4 mg; Syp 2, 4 mg/5 ml; MDI 100 mcg/puff; Rotacap 200 mcg/cap; Respule 2.5 mg/3 ml
Montelukast	2–5 yrs: 4 mg HS 6–14 yrs: 5 mg HS > 14 yrs: 10 mg HS	—	Tab 4, 5, 10 mg

(Contd.)

Drug	Dose	Maximum dose	Formulation
Levosalbutamol	Dose is ½ of salbutamol	—	Tab 1, 2 mg; Syp 0.5, 1 mg/5 ml; Respules 0.63, 1.25 mg
Salmeterol	50–100 mcg/d BD	—	MDI 25, 50 mcg/puff; Rotacap 50 mcg/cap
Terbutaline	0.1–0.15 mg/kg/d TDS oral 0.005–0.01 mg/kg/dose q 4 hrly SC 0.4–1 (max 10) mcg/kg/min IV 1–2 puffs QID; *Nebulisation:* 2.5 mg (< 20 kg); 5 mg(> 20 kg)	—	Tab 2.5, 5 mg; Syp 1.5/5 ml, 2.5/10 ml; Inj 0.5 mg/ml; MDI 250 mcg/puff; Neb sol 10 mg/ml
HORMONES			
Deflazacort	0.25–1.5 mg/kg/d BD/TDS	—	Tab 1, 6, 30 mg
Dexamethasone	*Anti-inflammatory action:* 0.05 mg/kg/dose QID; *CAH (Congenital adrenal hyperplasia):* 0.5–1 mg/d (oral) *Cerebral edema:* 0.5 mg/kg/dose QID; *Hib meningitis:* 0.15 mg/kg/dose QID; *Autoimmune disorders (Pulse therapy):* 5 mg/kg as a slow infusion (max 100 mg)	—	Tab 0.5 mg; Inj 4 mg/ml
Hydrocortisone	Anti-inflammatory: 2.5–10 mg/kg/d QID Status asthmaticus: 10 mg/kg/d stat f/b 5 mg/kg/dose QID IV Endotoxic shock: 50 mg/kg stat f/b 50–150 mg/kg d QID for 48–72 hrs IV Acute adrenal insufficiency: 50 mg/sq. m/d IV initially f/b 100 mg/sq. m/d (long-term replacement 10 mg/sq. m/d) CAH (Initial) 10–15 mg/sq. m/d (1/4 morning – 1/4 morning – 1/2 evening) Maintainance 0.3–0.4 mg/kg/d (div. as above)	—	Tab 5, 10, 20 mg; Inj 100 mg/vial
Methylprednisolone	0.4–1.7 mg/kg/d IM/IV/oral Pulse therapy: 30 mg/kg for 3–5 days Shock: 30 mg/kg/dose QID for 2–3 days	—	Tab 4, 8, 16 mg; Inj Solumedrol 140, 500 mg, 1, 2 gm vials; Inj Depomedrol 40 mg/ml
Prednisolone	1–2 mg/kg/d TDS	—	Tab 5, 10, 20, 30, 40; Syp 5 mg/5 ml, 10 mg/5 ml; 15 mg/5 ml

(Contd.)

Drug	Dose	Maximum dose	Formulation
ACTH	Anti-inflammatory: 0.8–1.6 U/kg/ IM or IV single dose Infantile spasms: 20–40 IU/kg/d IM BD	100 IU	20 IU/ml, 40 IU/ml, 80 IU/ml, 250 IU/ml
Desmopressin	Diabetes insipidus (Intranasal): 5–30 mcg OD/BD (Oral): 0.05 mg/dose BD (max 0.8 mg) Primary nocturnal enuresis; 20 mcg/d (max 40 mcg) [never use for > 28 days] IM/IV 4 mcg	—	Tab 0.1, 0.2 mg; 10 mcg/spray; Inj 4 mcg/ml; DDAVP 100 mcg/ml
Somatotropin (hGH)	0.18–0.3 mg/kg/week SC till desired height achieved/epiphyseal fusion occurs; For Turner's: 0.375 mg/kg/week	—	Inj 4, 10, 12, 16 IU 1 mg = 3 IU
Vasopressin	DI: 5–20 u q 4 hr SC/IM CDI: 1.5–10 mu/kg/min Variceal bleeding: 0.33/kg over 15 min f/b 0.33 u/kg/hr Shock: 0.3–2 mu/kg/min	—	Inj 20 u/ml
Propylthiouracil	1–4 mg/kg/d < 10 yrs: 50–150 mg/d TDS > 10 yrs: 150–300 mg/d TDS	—	Tab 50 mg
Thyroxine	NB: 10–15 mcg/kg/d; Children: 5 mcg/kg/d (empty stomach)	—	Tab 25, 50, 100, 200 mcg

TRANQUILLISERS, SEDATIVES, HYPNOTICS & ANTI-DEPRESSANTS			
Amitriptyline	Depression: 1 mg/kg/d BD (max 1.5 mg/kg) PNE: < 12 yrs: 10–25 mg HS > 12 yrs: 25–50 mg HS (for 8 weeks) Migraine prophylaxis: 0.1–0.25 mg/kg/dose HS (may increase by 0.25 mg/kg/ dose weekly (max. 2 mg/kg dose)	—	Tab 10, 25, 50, 75 mg
Atomoxetine	0.5 mg/kg/d (may be increased to max. 1.2 mg/kg) C/I < 6 yrs	—	Tab 10, 18, 25, 40 mg
Imipramine	PNE (> 6 yrs): Start with 10–25 mg HS (increase by 10–25 mg every 1–2 weeks until the desired effect, continue for 2–3 mths then taper. When dry for 2 consecutive weeks give EOD for next 2 weeks 6–12 yrs: 50 mg/d 12–14 yrs: 75 mg/d	—	Tab 25 mg, 75 mg

(Contd.)

Drug	Dose	Maximum dose	Formulation
Ketamine	Minor procedures: 0.5–1 mg/kg; sedative dose 2 mg/kg. Continuous infusion: 5–20 mcg/kg/min (sedation in ventilated pts)	—	Inj 10 mg/ml; 50 mg/ml
Trichlorophos	20 mg/kg/dose for sedation	—	Syp 500 mg/5 ml
Clonidine	Narcotic withdrawl (NB): 1–2 mcg/kg/dose TDS (max 2 mcg/kg/dose 4 hrly) ADHD: 0.05 mg/d (increase by 0.05 mg every 3–7 days max 0.4 mg/d QID [taper gradually]	—	Tab 100 mcg
Haloperidol	Chorea: 0.01–0.03 mg/kg/d BD/TDS Infantile autism: 0.025–0.05 mg/kg/d BD/TDS Psychotic disorder: 0.05–0.15 mg/kg/d BD/TDS Non-psychotic behaviour disorder: 0.05–0.075 mg/kg/d BD/TDS Gilles de la tourette syndrome: 0.05–0.075 mg/kg/d BD/TDS	—	Tab 0.25, 1.5, 5, 10, 20 mg
Nitrazepam	0.5–1 mg/kg/d BD	—	Tab 5, 10 mg

VITAMINS & HEMATINICS

Drug	Dose	Maximum dose	Formulation
Folic acid	0.5–1 mg/d for 4 wks f/b 200 mcg/d	—	Tab 5 mg
Iron	Prophylaxis: 3 mg/kg/d Treatment: 6 mg/kg/d	—	Syp 250/5 ml; 30, 60 mg/5 ml; Drops 25 mg/ml
Vitamin A	Oral: < 6 mths: 50000 IU 6–12 mths:1 lac IU > 12 mths: 2 lac IU IV: half of oral Prophlaxis: at 9 mths, 18 mths then every 6 mthly till 3 yrs of age Treatment: same dose at day 0, 1 and 4 weeks	—	Cap 25000 IU/cap; Inj 50000 IU/ml
Vitamin B_{12}	250–1000 mcg every alternate days for 1–2 weeks, then weekly until counts are normal; Maintenance: 1000 mcg every 2–4 mthly	—	Inj 1000 mcg/2 ml (with B_1 and B_6)
Pyridoxine	Prevention of INH neuropathy: 10 mg/d Treatment of INH neuropathy: 50 mg TDS Pyridoxine dependent seizures: 100 mg IV over 1 min (maximum 400 mg) F/B oral 50–100 mg/d	—	Tab 40 mg, 100 mg; Inj 100 mg/ml

(Contd.)

Drug	Dose	Maximum dose	Formulation
Vitamin C	100–300 mg/d oral/IV	—	Tab 200, 500 mg; Drops 100 mg/ml; Inj 500 mg/5 ml
Vitamin D₃	Treatment of rickets: 60000 IU/d oral for 10 days or 6 lac IU IM single dose	—	Sachet 60000 IU/sachet Inj 3 lac, 6 lac IU/ml
Vitamin E	Neonates: 25–35 IU/d Children: 1 IU/kg/d Sickle cell anemia: 450 IU/d Beta thalessemia: 750 IU/d Cystic fibrosis: 100–400 IU/d	—	Evion pearls 30, 100, 200, 400, 600 mg; Evion drops 50 mg/ml (1 mg = 1 IU)

MISCELLANEOUS			
Acetazolamide	Diuretic: 5 mg/kg/d TDS Hydrocephalus: 610 mg/kg/d TDS	—	Tab 250 mg
Albumin	0.5–1 g/kg over 2–4 hrs (rapidly in shock)	6 g/kg in 24 hrs	5% 250 ml, 500 ml; 20% 50 ml, 100 ml
Allopurinol	10 mg/kg/d TDS	600 mg	Tab 100, 300 mg
Baclofen	0.75–2 mg/kg/d TDS	< 8 yrs: 40 mg/d > 8 yrs: 60 mg/d	Tab 10, 25 mg
Betahistine	8–16 mg thrice a day Avoid < 12 yrs	75 mg/d	Tab 8, 16, 24 mg
Caffeine	20 mg/kg (L) over 20 min f/b 5 mg/kg (M) OD (IV/oral)	—	Inj/oral 20 mg/ml
Calcium gluconate	1–2 ml/kg/dose stat; 1 ml/kg/dose QID	—	10% calcium gluconate contains 100 mg/ml of Ca gluconate i.e. 8.9 mg/ml elemental Ca or Ca ionic 0.45 meq/ml
Deferipone	50–100 mg/kg/d BD	—	250, 500 tab
Dextromethorphan	1–2 mg/kg/d TDS	—	Syp 30 mg/5 ml 10 mg/ 5 ml
Flunarizine	5 mg/d (only > 5 yrs)	—	Tab 5, 10 mg
Lactulose	1–2 ml/kg/d QID	—	—
Lanzoperazole	1 mg/kg/d OD	—	Tab 15 mg
Mannitol	5 ml/kg f/b 2 ml/kg QID or 0.5–3 g/kg/dose TDS	—	—

(Contd.)

Drug	Dose	Maximum dose	Formulation
Methotrexate	5–10 mg/sq metre empty stomach once weekly	—	Tab 2.5, 5, 7.5 mg
Methylphenidate	0.3–1 mg/kg/d (start with 5 mg before BF and lunch increase by 5–10 mg/week	2 mg/kg/d or 60 mg/d	Ritalin 5, 10, 20 mg Avoid < 6 yrs; ADHD
Piracetam	40 mg/kg/d TDS	—	Cap 400, 800 mg; Syp 500/5 ml
Racecodotril	1.5 mg/kg/dose TDS	—	Sach 10, 30 mg; Cap 100 mg
Ranitidine	1–2 mg/kg/d BD IV	—	—
Sod. bicarbonate	1–2 mEq/kg or calculate as 0.6* base deficit* weight	—	0.9 mEq/ml amp (10 ml)
Ursedeoxycholic acid	10–15 mg/kg/d TDS	—	Tab 150, 250, 300 mg
Zinc	< 6 mths – 10 mg/d > 6 mths – 20 mg/d Acrodermatitis enteropathica – 6 mg/kg/d	—	Syp 20 mg/5 ml; Drops 2.5 mg/ml

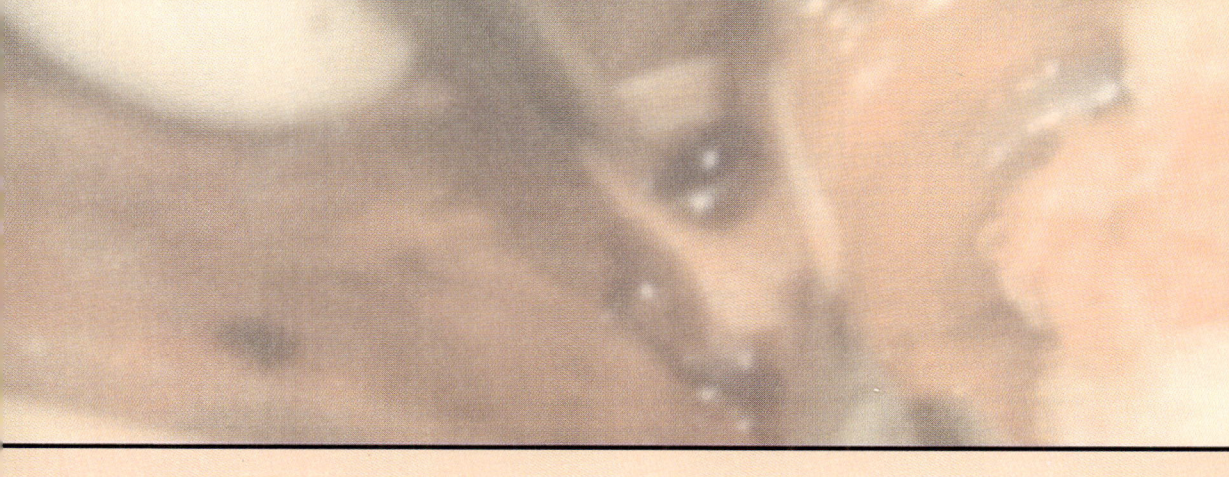

Index